Media Literacy and Mental Health Care Access

Media Literacy and Mental Health Care Access

Jesse Scaccia

BLOOMSBURY ACADEMIC
NEW YORK • LONDON • OXFORD • NEW DELHI • SYDNEY

BLOOMSBURY ACADEMIC
Bloomsbury Publishing Inc
Bloomsbury Publishing Inc, 1385 Broadway, New York, NY 10018, USA
Bloomsbury Publishing Plc, 50 Bedford Square, London, WC1B 3DP, UK
Bloomsbury Publishing Ireland, 29 Earlsfort Terrace, Dublin 2, D02 AY28, Ireland

First published in the United States of America 2026

A catalog record for this book is available from the Library of Congress

ISBN: HB: 978-1-6669-6509-4
ePDF: 979-8-2162-6386-9
eBook: 978-1-9787-6286-2

Typeset by Deanta Global Publishing Services, Chennai, India

To the professionals who help young adults reach the mental health care they need, including mental health care promoters, providers, and everyone who teaches young adults the skills they use to access this care.

And to the folks who supported me and believed in me leading up to and through this process, including Mike Humphrey, Jessie Tepper, Alicia Cintron, Faith Sidlow, Kathleen Chavoor, and my cat, Pippin.

Finally, to my wonderful family and to the mental health care professionals who helped me become the kind of person capable of completing a project like this.

Contents

Introduction

On October 13, 2023, California governor Gavin Newsom signed into law Assembly Bill 873, mandating the integration of media literacy instruction into the four core subjects that all students learn from kindergarten through twelfth grade in California ("California to Teach Media Literacy in Every Grade" 2023). California has the largest public school system in America, with almost six million students, making this a very big deal in the world of media literacy education (National Center for Education Statistics 2024). According to the text of the bill, "It is therefore the intent of the Legislature to ensure that all pupils in California are prepared with media literacy skills necessary to safely, responsibly, and critically consume and use social media and other forms of media" ("Bill Text—AB-873 Pupil Instruction: Media Literacy" 2024).

California isn't the only state mandating media literacy education in its public schools. Other large states like Texas and Florida, along with eighteen other states, mandated some version of media literacy education in their schools as of May 2024 (Media Literacy Now 2024). "Media literacy" is a malleable concept, leading to a cornucopia of pedagogical directions cited in the bills. Florida emphasized digital wellness, telling teachers to educate students on the ways social media can negatively impact their mental health (Johnson 2024). New Jersey focused on "information literacy," which it defined as "a set of skills that enables an individual to recognize when information is needed and to locate, evaluate, and effectively use the needed information" (Office of the Governor 2023). The New Mexico state government is looking to instill digital citizenship practices and foster skills like the reporting of cyberbullying and online reputation management (New Mexico Public Education Department 2024).

Media literacy is a concept not unlike putty that can be formed into almost infinite shapes. There are dozens of ways that public school systems and universities currently implementing media literacy education can define and operationalize the term. Yes, our students need to understand how social media is impacting them, and yes, we need to be training skillful and thoughtful digital citizens so they can be good citizens. But as battles rage across the headlines and around the world, the most immediate battles facing young adults in America are the wars within themselves.

The kids are not alright, and they're not accessing the care they need. Young adults in the United States aged eighteen to twenty-nine have the highest lifetime rates of depression diagnoses, with 34.3 percent reporting they have been diagnosed, compared with much lower rates among those over forty-four (Gallup 2023). Almost one in five young adults (eighteen to twenty-five years old) experienced a major depressive episode in the past year (National Institute of Mental Health 2024), yet the majority of young adults with depression don't get help (Wang et al. 2022). And that doesn't include other forms of mental health issues.

Media literacy courses teaching students how news, media, and social media might cause or worsen their mental health are a start. This book makes the case that media literacy education also needs to teach young adults how to reach that help. Today and into the future, media is the pathway that leads those in need of care to the care available to them, in many cases. This part of the access to mental health care ecosystem is what this project is seeking to tease out. How do young adults want to receive information about available mental health care services? What role does and can various forms of media play in making mental health care more accessible?

Our young people *want* media literacy education; they're just not all getting it. Ninety-four percent of young people wish their schools taught media literacy, but only 39 percent received such instruction during the 2023–4 school year, according to a 2024 online survey of 1,110 teens ages 13–18 (News Literacy Project 2024). It feels inevitable that media literacy education will continue to spread across America, like a ripple on a flag, and the timing is perfect. With the rapid decline of local newspapers (Medill Local News Initiative 2023) and the rapid diffusion of ways media can reach us through technology (Lee and Smith 2023), our society needs to re-learn how to communicate with itself. This includes those promoting available mental health care options and the many of us desperate to be reached.

I was only forty-five years old at the time of this writing, yet I remember when the doctor would send you a letter, you would read that letter because letters were a big deal. What's the best way to reach today's young adults with information about the mental health care options available to them? Do they want to be YouTube'd, Snapchatted, or do they want to receive this information more innocuously, like through billboards or newsletters? What role should face-to-face promotion of mental health options play? We can improve the mental health of our young people by building smarter connective tissue, or pathways, between those in need and the health care that's out there for them. And media literacy skills give young adults the tools and confidence to navigate those pathways.

With better maps and better map readers, we can increase mental health care access.

* * *

The motivation for this book is personal. For much of my upbringing, I suffered from a basket of mental health conditions, including diagnoses of major depression, complex post-traumatic stress disorder (PTSD), anxiety, and suggestions of borderline personality disorder. While I have always been ahead of the curve in terms of both literacy and personal empowerment, I failed to get the help I needed for decades. These untreated conditions negatively impacted my career, made it hard to maintain relationships, and kept me on the edge of suicidality for most of my adult life. I broke my family's heart too many times with late-night calls asking them to please just let me go, so I could be done with the pain.

I needed help. I knew I needed help. Help, in various forms, was out there. Over time, I had various insurance plans, and at times I was eligible for public care. But help wasn't reaching me—at least not in a way that I *heard*

In retrospect, I cannot help but wonder where the disconnect was. I was as media-obsessed as any young adult. What medium would I have been receptive to? What rhetoric and messaging? What would the map have looked like that led me from the dark pit I was in to a new reality of hope and healing?

When I was thirty-nine years old, I went back to school to get my PhD. During this time, I committed to myself to fix the mental and physical health issues that had long felt like yolks on my shoulders. Going back to school, I learned communication theories and more about how our brains process information and emotion, but I also gained a new sense of empowerment toward increasing my own health and mental health efficacies. I learned there were more options than just cognitive behavioral therapy. I learned there were somatic therapeutic modalities that could help heal the heart and soul. I experienced therapy in person, online, solo, and in groups. I learned about which therapies worked for the different aspects of trauma and self that I needed to heal. I was, finally, *reached.*

I almost, or could have, died as a result of the symptom of suicidality, as so many men in our country do, with rates 3.85 times higher than those of women (American Foundation for Suicide Prevention 2024). Media literacy education, more effective mental health care messaging, and greater personal mental health literacy (MHL) could have saved me sooner, I'm convinced.

This research is for younger me, and my current and future students. In most of my classes, I encourage writing in the first-person perspective. My students improve as writers by honing their own stories. Through this, I get to know the young adults that pass through my classroom quite well. I don't just see them in action; I'm afforded access to their inner worlds and thoughts. While the young adults in my classes are bright, loving, and wise beyond their years, so many of them are lonely. So many of them have crushing anxiety. So many of them have gone through things in the past that still greatly impact them today, affecting their classroom performances, their ability to make connections, and their sense of hope.

Personally, I suffered from mental health issues before the Internet, so I can't blame social media or the 24/7 news cycle or the COVID-19 global pandemic for being the root cause of my mental illness. While depression has potentially always existed (Jackson 2024), what's changed rapidly is the conversation around mental health and mental health care, and the role media has come to play as a mediator to accessing mental health care. If mental health care is the Emerald City, the messaging that leads a young adult from where they are to care is their Yellow Brick Road.

They have to know the care exists. They have to be drawn to it with the right messaging. They have to know they're safe to get care. So many of them need help. And help is available to many of them, for free, from student health centers and community clinics. But the majority of them don't get the help they need, help that's just a call or a click away.

Where's the disconnect? How can we do better?

Let's dive in and find out.

To better understand what's going on here, we will start with a chapter that dives into the latest research and best practices about getting the word out about available mental health care services, or more broadly put, health promotion messaging. In Chapter 2, I provide an overview of the current state of mental health of young adults, what we know about their barriers to accessing mental health care, and the role the media (and social media) is playing in our young adults' mental health. Chapter 3 will help the reader better understand the media literacy movement: where did it come from, how state departments of education are implementing new media literacy policies passed by state assemblies, and what the research is telling us about how media literacy-centered interventions are helping people become more empowered citizens and healthier humans. Although a number of international studies are referenced, the research cited in these sections primarily centers on an American context. This emphasis reflects the book's objective: to inform and support US policy, mental health care systems, and the experiences of young adults in the United States.

Chapters 4 and 5 include original research. I interviewed thirty young adults in California's Central Valley to better understand how they want to receive information about available mental health care services. Which media and mediums do they trust the most? Which storytellers and methods of storytelling? How do they envision the ideal bridge of information between young adults in need and the care out there waiting for them? Then, I interviewed twenty mental health care providers and promoters in the Central Valley, seeking to uncover the media literacy expectations mental health care providers and promoters have for the young adults seeking care in their community. What media are mental health care promoters and providers using? What's the pathway where those providing and needing care can meet in the middle?

In the conclusion, I bring together the existing research, the voices of young adults, and the insights of mental health care professionals to draw conclusions and make recommendations. I have a few audiences in mind for these recommendations: legislators who make media literacy education policy, media literacy educators whose job it is to teach those policies, and mental health care promoters, with student health centers especially in mind.

A quick note on my approach. In doing the research for this book, I highly privileged studies conducted since 2020, with much of the research conducted in the last two years. The COVID-19 global pandemic changed things. Media keeps changing. The fresher the research, the better with a topic like this. I favored studies with large sample sizes that took place over multiple years. I also drew from an international array of researchers and institutions. I tried to include as many meta-analyses—when a researcher looks at all the research on a topic, finds a way to combine the data or findings, and summarizes where the literature as a whole is at—as possible. Beyond just parenthetical citations, I try to include a little more about the study so readers can draw some of their own conclusions about how applicable findings would be in their community or with a population that they serve.

While the goal of this research is to lead to findings that are generalizable across young adult populations, I am also openly invested in the mental health of the young adults in the Central Valley and at Fresno State, so the research cited is sometimes centered in this diverse and bountiful part of the world.

"Our system of mental health care in California falls short, not for lack of funding," said Governor Newsom (Botts et al. 2024). "We've done the right thing in this state . . . we passed a millionaire's tax in 2004 that now funnels more than $2 billion a year into services. We fall short because we lack the bold leadership and strategic vision necessary to bring the most advanced forms of care to scale across the state."

I believe that helping more of our young adults get the care they need for their depression, anxiety, and other mental illnesses is well within our reach. The aim is that the research collected in this book is a small step toward a more efficient and humane model of disseminating information about available care.

1

Getting the Good Word Out

Health Promotion Messaging in the Contemporary Era

A little more than ten years ago, Lisa Sontag-Padilla and her team collected an illuminating data set about California college students' experiences receiving information related to mental health and available mental health care services (Sontag-Padilla et al. 2018). Over 19,900 students across thirty campuses completed both parts of the survey. The research focused on campuses that had already spent a year implementing campus-based California Mental Health Services Authority grants to enhance prevention and early intervention activities for student mental health. These campuses had the support to do more, and still, just over half of students—56.6 percent—said they were aware of where to go on campus if they needed mental health or similar supportive services.

"Our findings call attention to the need for more-efficient methods of disseminating information about mental health services and topics to students," Sontag and her team wrote (Sontag-Padilla et al. 2018). While their findings are relatively dated, it is data that is available that most directly sets the stage for this chapter. Neither this team nor anyone else seems to have replicated a similar study since, at least that I found, so I can't say for sure how much the 56.6 percent statistic has changed. Yet, the call still rings out to get more effective at reaching college students—and all young adults—with information about the mental health care available to them.

These findings are reflected in the even larger Healthy Minds Study, which polled 76,406 college students across more than 200 universities (Healthy Minds Network 2023). When asked for their response to the statement, "If I needed to seek professional help for my mental or emotional health, I would know where to go to access resources from my school," only 46 percent of students agreed or strongly agreed. If our college students, who should have both higher literacy than their peers and greater access to mental health care, don't know where to get care, it becomes essential to understand how this communication breakdown can be fixed.

In this chapter, I examine what we know works when it comes to reaching people with information about mental health care. I start with a few theoretical models of health promotion and behavior change to set the stage for the chapter and the original research later in this book that is built off those theories. I then look into what the research has taught us about the intersection between health promotion and social media, and the mediums young adults are using to access information about mental health care. Finally, I dive into the literature to see what I find in terms of best practices for reaching people with information about mental health care.

A common refrain was found among discussion sections of articles related to these topics: further qualitative research is warranted to obtain a more nuanced understanding of how media impacts the general public's decision to seek help for mental illness (Goodwin and Behan 2023).

The marketing and promotion of mental health options is the bridge between need and care. The more members of the community make it over that bridge early in their mental illness, the better. Preventing mental disorders depends on people with early symptoms seeking help from professionals for diagnosis or treatment (Michel et al. 2018). Understanding the communication that facilitates care—and the barriers to seeking help—is crucial for facilitating care early on after the onset of mental illness.

Theories of Behavior Change and Models of Health Communication

Decades of usage by both academics and professional communicators have led to durable behavior change theories that are relevant to this conversation and research.

This research is grounded in the Theory of Planned Behavior (TPB; Ajzen 1985). The TPB model posits that the intent to engage in a behavior is the primary determinant of behavior. This intent is impacted by three factors: perceived social norms about the action; attitude toward the action; and whether or not individuals think they can successfully complete the behavior, or self-efficacy. In this research, I am focused on the media literacy efficacies expected by mental health practitioners and administrators of young adults seeking mental health care. I am also interested in determining the existing media literacy efficacies of young adults so that communicators of mental health opportunities can reach young adults through media channels with messaging that is most appealing to them.

TPB is used to guide the structure of research, as it does here, in which a section of questions mirrors its three predeterminations of intent. Its validity also appears organically in research results. A study from the Amsterdam Public Health Institute tracked young adults and adolescents who found their way to mental health care to treat their depression symptoms (Eigenhuis et al. 2021). Three of the top four themes identified among those who had made it to professional help were in line with TPB: individual functioning (efficacy), attitude, and surroundings—with health literacy the fourth most common theme.

Social Cognitive Theory (SCT), which is also commonly used in health communication research and is closely related to TPB, also guided this research. A foundational concept of SCT is reciprocal determinism, which explains that human behavior is influenced by personal factors (i.e., beliefs, attitudes, and knowledge), behavior (i.e., practices and actions of the individual), and environmental factors (social norms, physical setting, external feedback; Bandura 1986).

This research also leans on trusted communication models like the Health Belief Model (HBM), which states that an individual's health-related behavior is determined by three factors: perception of threat of the health problem, benefits of avoiding the problem, and the barriers to taking action (Hochbaum 1958). A lack of the functional media literacy skills necessary to access mental health care is one of the barriers to taking action I am attempting to tackle here.

Mental Health Care Promotion for Young Adults

"Understanding the risk factors and triggers for mental health problems in young adults is crucial," wrote Caroline Mitchell, a British GP and researcher, and their team, "however we also need to know more about how young adults seek help, if we wish to improve the quality and outcomes of mental health care" (Mitchell et al. 2017, 8). These authors make key points that help us understand when and if a young adult will seek care: just because a young adult knows they have a problem and has access to care does not mean they will access that care, and the roles and concerns of family, tutors, peers, and employers play a significant role in whether a young adult makes their way to care.

It probably isn't surprising to learn that the vast majority of young adults (aged 18–25) use their mobile phones to look online for help for a personal or emotional concern, with over 80 percent of them indicating this, as part of an Irish survey of 1,308 respondents (Pretorius et al. 2019). A similar percentage of young adults went straight to an Internet search for help, while 57 percent went to a health website, according to the same study. Young adults were drawn to the anonymity and confidentiality offered by the Internet, but then often found the reliability of the resources unclear. Things that made them trust online mental health resources more included a health service logo and endorsements from schools or colleges.

Led by Pretorius and their team, the aforementioned Irish researcher looked at how digital pathways best create ways to help for young people (Pretorius et al. 2020). They identified four key design considerations: connectedness, accessible information, personalization, and immediacy. They urged mental health care communicators to build trust into their communication in actionable ways. "Helping young people to assign credibility to online resources also has the potential to play an important role in developing their mental health literacy," they wrote (Pretorius et al. 2020, 5). "The findings from the survey indicate that young people value information that is backed by research and written by experts in the field. Young people's online information-gathering behaviours can be facilitated by including hyperlinks to other online resources that can complement the help-seeking journey." They also stressed the importance of developing messaging that is conscious of different kinds of help-seekers, as each mental health condition comes with its own set of barriers.

The framing of care is critical to reach young adults seeking mental health help online. An Australian research team conducted a mixed methods study examining young people's attitudes toward help sources and how receptive young people are to the influence of others on their help-seeking intentions (Stretton et al. 2018). They found that young people need marketing to be clear about what help services offer, how they treat mental health concerns, and what an individual can expect when seeking support online. When services and systems are complex and the barriers are many, it's not enough to offer care. A detailed look at that care should be provided as well.

Social support is a major determinant of whether young adults have a positive attitude about seeking mental health care, found a Canadian study designed to examine help-seeking preferences among 167 first-year university students (Samuel and Kamenetsky 2022). In a related finding from the same study, students were most inclined to seek support from informal sources and least inclined to seek support from formal sources. Students were equally likely to seek support from friends, family, and the Internet. These factors create a unique challenge for those promoting their organization's mental health care services: how does an organization promote its services when that organization is seen as a less attractive messenger?

Generally speaking, media mental health awareness campaigns are associated with positive changes in attitudes, beliefs, and intentions, as well as positive changes in behaviors, including increased help-seeking among people aged ten to twenty-four (Tam et al. 2024). Tam and their Vancouver-based team looked at fifteen campaigns from eight different countries, with campaigns disseminated through television, webpages, billboards, print ads, and social media platforms such as Twitter, Facebook, and YouTube. "The results demonstrate the potential of utilizing media campaigns as a tool for mental health promotion, particularly for a youth demographic group," the authors wrote (Tam et al. 2024, 918), along with a note of caution that these campaigns should be continually and rigorously evaluated.

Wright and their team looked at twenty-seven studies related to mental health digital interventions directed toward those eleven to eighteen years old (Wright et al. 2023). They called the effects found across the studies small but promising, noting improvements in help-seeking behaviors, with outcomes shaped by factors such as support networks and the setting in which care was sought. They point to future research that better examines how diversity-sensitive design and content mediates and facilitates the path to mental health care.

People who experience mental illness often demonstrate limited help-seeking behaviors, as Goodwin and Behan noted in their review of how media impacts help-seeking behaviors (Goodwin and Behan 2023). Across the sixteen studies, they found that various forms of media—including video and online resources—can positively influence help-seeking for mental health, with print media having a much more limited effect. The authors found notable promise in video as a connector at multiple stops along the pathway of care. Their review pointed toward the potency of video-based interventions that could both impact attitudes and have the potential to encourage people to access professional help.

The impact of print media that promotes mental health options has a particularly dulled effect on young people, found a large trial in British schools (Sharpe et al. 2017). There was no detectable impact of booklets on mental health, quality of life, or help-seeking, the researchers found, in results supported by the work of an Indian team who found that young people could not recall information about mental health resources shared through print media (Shrivastava et al. 2014).

Other meta-analyses have similarly demonstrated that, although all help-seeking campaigns yielded improvements in at least one help-seeking outcome, those employing traditional methods have been less effective (Johnson et al. 2021). Studies aimed at improving mental health literacy (MHL) and help-seeking by utilizing mediums such as emails, posters, campus programs, and so on, have shown no significant changes in help-seeking intention or behavior (Reavley et al. 2014). This could be due to the intervention's promotive and informational nature and lack of personalized components (Johnson et al. 2021).

Web-based campaigns seem to be more effective among young adults, as online delivery of care, participant involvement, and embedded links to professional services were all found to encourage help-seeking (Johnson et al. 2021). Among the outcomes this Indian team studied, help-seeking attitude was seen as the most malleable outcome of the intervention, followed by help-seeking intention (Johnson et al. 2021). The more those elements can be tailored to specific audiences, the better they can increase the effectiveness of help-seeking campaigns (Johnson et al. 2020).

Young adults don't just want mental health care delivered through technology; they also want mental health care outreach to be delivered through technology (Liu and Zhang 2024). This research team, researching out of the University of Texas at Austin, also found that digital mental health promotion can act as a valuable stopping point on the way to other mental health resources, with technology providing basic knowledge and emotional preparation before, say, meeting with a counselor in the embodied world.

Digital mental health care promotion attempting to reach young people should emphasize that patients—and what they share—will be kept anonymous (Garrido et al. 2022). These Australian researchers found that young people want to feel empowered to make their own decisions about accessing professional help, and that directive language can act as a deterrent to accessing care.

There is a risk that mental health promotion campaigns may unintentionally cause harm. For instance, campaigns aimed at addressing suicidality can inadvertently increase perceptions that suicidal behavior is common or frequent (Niederkrotenthaler et al. 2014). As outlined by the guiding theories of this book—including TFB—social norms are a key determinant of behavior. Thus, anti-suicide campaigns "may increase the likelihood that individuals will believe that engaging in suicidal behavior is widespread and therefore acceptable" (Niederkrotenthaler et al. 2014, S235).

Care Through Media

A number of major factors have converged in recent years to make online mental health care a viable option for more people, including the COVID-19 global pandemic lockdowns and the manifold spread of digital tools, such as Zoom and the improvement of video cameras on phones. The cost-effectiveness, anonymity, accessibility, and adaptability are also attractive features (Wright et al. 2023), lowering the threshold to care (Mrazek et al. 2019). "It now seems inevitable that digital technologies will change the face of mental health research and treatment," wrote Torous and their team in their analysis of the future of digital psychiatry (Torous et al. 2021, 330). "The extent to which these changes are genuinely beneficial for those with mental disorders will depend on equitable access, robust research, and ethical, evidence-based implementation of these new technologies within global mental health care," they concluded.

Digital mental health interventions can be effective, with studies showing variable rates of success. While it may be attractive to embrace virtual mental health care as a more convenient one-for-one alternative to the face-to-face care that has been the hallmark of mental health care interventions since, arguably, the beginning of human history, the experts are not all quite there yet. A 2019 meta-analysis looked at forty-eight studies that examined Internet mental health interventions for college students (Harrer et al. 2019). The authors found small effects for depression, anxiety, and stress, with more robust effects for eating disorders and role functioning. A 2022 meta-analysis—focused on all people, not just college students—showed online interventions significantly prevent an increase in depression scores but not in stress and anxiety scores (Noh and Kim 2023). Another 2022 meta-analysis of digital health interventions for the delivery of mental health care looked at 304 studies and concluded that virtual reality, mobile apps, social media platforms, and web-based forums are novel technologies that have the potential to improve mental health but require higher quality evidence (Philippe et al. 2022).

Greenwood and their team's 2022 analysis looked at cognitive behavioral and family therapies delivered in populations encompassing addiction disorders, eating disorders, childhood mental health problems, and chronic conditions (Greenwood et al. 2022). Their study of over twelve randomized controlled trials, including 931 patients, found there was insufficient evidence of a difference between psychotherapy delivered via telehealth and the same therapy delivered face-to-face. From the perspective of this research, there is graceful efficiency in young adults learning about available care online and then receiving said care through the same device (which they already possess and know how to use). It reduces the amount of effort needed to access and act on care.

Smartphone applications (apps) hold promise as a stand-alone self-management tool in mental health service delivery, found Leech and their team out of Australia, who looked at eleven randomized controlled trials and a pooled sample of 1,706 adolescents and young adults ranging in age from ten to thirty-five years old (Leech et al. 2021). App interventions produced significant symptom improvement across multiple outcomes compared to waitlist or attention control conditions, they found. They pointed to apps as a good opportunity for young adults to learn vital mental health and wellness skills, such as mindfulness.

Bantjes (2022) built on these themes, noting that apps are uniquely positioned to overcome some of the challenges typically associated with providing adolescent mental health services, including scheduling problems, adolescents' reluctance to seek help from professionals, and their developmentally appropriate need for autonomy and independence (Bantjes 2022). They noted the power of the relative anonymity(of getting care through an app versus face-to-face), which is a way to circumvent stigma and give the individual more of a sense of control over what is a stressful process for many, even in the best of situations. These interventions may work for some conditions better than others. As Lehtimaki and their team found in their analysis of eighteen studies, there is evidence to support the effectiveness of computerized cognitive behavioral therapy on anxiety and depression, whereas the effectiveness of other digital mental health interventions remains inconclusive (Lehtimaki et al. 2021).

Digital interventions work better than no intervention to improve depression in young people, according to a 2019 systematic analysis (Garrido et al. 2019). That said, these results are contingent on whether the digital care is highly supervised; and no matter the level of support, digital interventions do not work better than active alternatives. Digital health interventions to promote health and wellness among adolescents may be scalable in community mental health settings, found a 2019 study (Aschbrenner et al. 2019). These researchers also emphasized the need for adult monitoring and support and suggested that digital health interventions for this group should focus on existing strengths and online peer support for health promotion. Peer support is identified as a facilitator of good digital care throughout the literature, including by Thomson and their team, who found that peer support can open up members to different types of experiences, build a support network, and improve symptoms (Thomson et al. 2024). A review of peer support similarly found associations with improved mental health, including greater happiness, self-esteem, the development of effective coping strategies, and reductions in depression, loneliness, and anxiety.

Digital mental health interventions can work in partnership with in-person interventions by enhancing readiness for therapy. Jardine and their team looked at forty-five studies that addressed digital programs designed to increase engagement with further psychological treatment (Jardine et al. 2022). Components of the interventions included psychoeducation, symptom assessment and feedback, information on treatment options and referrals, client testimonials, expectation management, and pro-con lists. But there are risks. While these programs are promising, "The complex nature of stigma, motivation, and individual emotional responses toward engaging in treatment for mental health difficulties suggests that a careful approach is needed when developing and evaluating digital readiness interventions," they wrote (Jardine et al. 2022, 1). It's easy to imagine someone who is already sensitive to the idea of mental health treatment being turned off by flat words on the digital page, without a trained human there to guide them through anxieties and misconceptions.

As artificial intelligence (AI) continues to improve, so will its ability to provide meaningful and nuanced feedback to patients, including mental health patients. AI can be implemented for a wide variety of purposes to support mental health identification, risk assessment, and treatment, according to a scoping review of artificial intelligence and machine learning in mobile apps for mental health (Milne-Ives et al. 2022). The authors noted that mobile devices can collect active data from participants and capture passive sensing data, providing a rich body of information for analysis and tailoring the provision of support.

Health Promotion and Social Media

Social media has made the world smaller, including reducing the distance between patients and health care systems. Physical barriers that traditionally impede access to health care resources and support are removed by social media, creating a whole new landscape compared to a generation ago. Today, it is difficult to imagine public health without social media, reported Dr. Michael Stellefson from the Department of Health Education and Promotion at East Carolina University and his team, in their article examining the updated responsibilities for health education specialists (Stellefson et al. 2020). "Social media provides an outlet to increase and promote translational health communication strategies and effective data dissemination, in ways that allow users to not only utilize but also create and share pertinent health information," they wrote (Stellefson et al. 2020, 5).

Mental health care providers don't have to hope a patient in need happens to take a bus that has an advertisement for services or see their advertisement on page B24 of the local paper. The marketing, and often the care, can more effectively than ever meet them where they are: scrolling. Stellefson and their team make clear that while social media won't be as effective in reaching older and less media-literate populations, young adults are reachable this way (Stellefson et al. 2020).

Michelle O'Reilly, a senior lecturer at the Greenwood Institute of Child Health, led a 2019 study that used focus groups to elicit opinions of fifty-four adolescents, sixteen educational professionals, and eight mental health practitioners regarding whether social media can be used to promote mental health to eleven to eighteen year olds (O'Reilly et al. 2019). They landed on three themes: social media appears to have the potential to promote positive mental health, adolescents frequently utilize social media and the Internet to seek information about mental health, and there are benefits and challenges to using social media in this way.

"Learning about mental health and illness through multiple platforms was important and (participants) argued that the Internet as an educational tool was valuable if used carefully and when supported by appropriate adults, such as teachers," the authors concluded (O'Reilly et al. 2019, 988). They suggested that while information should be shared through social media, it should be social media somehow curated by the school. They noted specific challenges to conveying mental health information through social media, including the credibility and trustworthiness of the sources of information. Adolescents want information quickly, and they "generally failed" to critically analyze information presented to them. Adolescents in their study cited visual media as preferable, such as Instagram and YouTube.

There is a distinction between providing mental health information—such as defining key terms, explaining therapeutic approaches, or demystifying mental health care systems—and actively promoting access to mental health care. While these areas are distinct, their intersection holds significant potential: when mental health information seamlessly connects users to accessible care, often just a click away, it amplifies both understanding and action.

Social media can be an effective way to reach people with information about mental health and mental health care, as Latha and their team found in a qualitative study of three health-related social media campaigns that reached over 10,000 people (Latha et al. 2020). Witnessing information about care is just one step along the road to care, but it's a critical one. There is no direct relationship between the shares, likes, and engagement shown on the social media pages and the actual behavioral change, they noted. Social media campaigns need to have a strong theoretical base—such as applying the TPB—to be effective (Freeman et al. 2015). And, of course, there are risks to health information being shared in real-time over social media, such as the lack of information gatekeepers facilitating the sharing of bad information (Qazvinian et al. 2011).

Social Media as a Direct Agent of Health Behavior Change

In the early 2010s, Facebook made headlines for using its powerful social media network to inspire the wrong kind of change in users: to make them less happy.

"For one week in January 2012, Facebook deliberately made about 155,000 people sad, just to see if it could," reported the *Guardian* (Hern 2014). Facebook experimented on nearly 700,000 newsfeeds—without the informed consent of users, a major ethical breach—hiding what they called a small percentage of emotional words from 0.04 percent of users' feeds. The silver lining of the questionable research method was interesting results. The study reinforced the validity of the concept of "emotional contagion," or the idea that "emotional states can be transferred to others via emotional contagion, leading people to experience the same emotions without their awareness," as defined by the authors, who included the Facebook data team and researchers from Cornell (Kramer et al. 2014, 8788–90). But what makes the Facebook study interesting is that in-person interaction and non-verbal cues are not necessary for emotions to jump from one person to another. Words on a screen attached to a name can be enough.

According to this research, to some degree, what social media users see, social media users do. When positive expressions were reduced, people produced fewer positive posts and more negative posts; when negative expressions were reduced, the opposite pattern occurred, the authors wrote (Kramer et al. 2014).

Social media can be harnessed to positively and effectively influence consumer behavior, encouraging choices that promote better health outcomes. These efforts are often referred to as Social Network Interventions (SNIs). Hunter et al. (2019) define SNIs as strategies that "specifically use or alter the characteristics of social networks to generate, accelerate, or maintain health behaviors." In their systematic review and meta-analysis of health behavior outcomes, Hunter and colleagues reported mixed findings. Interventions targeting sexual health outcomes showed effectiveness in both the short and long term. Similarly, interventions addressing well-being, smoking cessation, and alcohol misuse demonstrated significant positive effects. However, interventions aimed at reducing drug-related risks did not yield statistically significant results. These mixed findings are echoed in earlier research by Johns et al. (2017), who conducted a systematic review on the use of social media for health promotion. Their study found that while the inclusion of online social elements did not consistently enhance smoking cessation or weight loss in health campaigns, social media messaging did improve physical activity levels.

Mental Health Promotion and Men: Inviting Men to Care

Let's take a closer look at what is known about how specific groups access information regarding available mental health care. Research consistently shows that young men are less likely than their female peers to seek help for mental health challenges (Burke et al. 2022). This disparity is particularly concerning given that suicide rates among male adolescents are three times higher than those of their female counterparts (Calear et al. 2017). Given the pressing concern for this demographic, we will spend a little more time reviewing what the research has to teach us about successfully inviting men to mental health care opportunities.

Media-based mental health campaigns can significantly influence male help-seeking behaviors for mental health challenges, according to the findings of a 2024 Australian systematic review (Duthie et al. 2024). The analysis included twenty-two studies that evaluated the effectiveness of media-based campaigns aimed at improving male attitudes, beliefs, intentions, or behaviors related to mental health issues, distress, suicide, or self-harm. The authors concluded, "The evidence collectively suggests that campaigns targeting mental health or depression can positively influence male help-seeking, including having an immediate effect on actual help-seeking behaviors" (Duthie et al. 2024, 11).

The authors argue that effective messaging and delivery of mental health-related content for male audiences should align with men's communication preferences (Duthie et al. 2024). These strategies include using male or mixed-gender campaign imagery, testimonials, humor, and gain-framed messages that portray help-seeking as strong, brave, or courageous. Men prefer to see pathways to personal growth and support that honor their identities without judgment. This insight complements findings by Smith et al. (2008), who utilized TPBto explore psychological help-seeking among young adult males. Their research underscores the importance of meeting men within the framework of their traditional masculinity ideology. By avoiding the requirement for men to fundamentally alter their views on traditional masculinity to access care, these approaches reduce barriers to behavior change and promote engagement.

"Targeting adaptive masculine stereotypes, such as responsibility, and reframing help-seeking to align with male values (e.g., presenting it as a sign of strength) may have contributed to improvements in help-seeking behaviors," concluded Sagar-Ouriaghli and colleagues as a result of their British study focusing on male students (Sagar-Ouriaghli et al. 2020, 12). The narrative of care matters, especially to men. Male students are a "very high-risk group that is even more reluctant to seek help for mental health difficulties, placing them at high risk of suicide" (Sagar-Ouriaghli et al. 2020). Their focus groups revealed themes that male students considered important when designing male-friendly interventions that addressed mental health help-seeking. The main two themes were: (1) protecting male vulnerability and (2) providing a masculine narrative of help-seeking.

Similarly, themes of self-reliance and emotional control emerged from research on the Men's Stress Workshop, an eight-week gender-sensitive group treatment for men experiencing symptoms of depression. These findings further support the argument that framing mental health care as a means of enhancing traditional masculine traits can be an effective strategy for engaging men (Primack et al. 2010).

Yousaf, Popat, and Hunter quantified these findings, revealing that men's attitudes toward traditional masculinity norms account for 50 percent of the variability in psychological help-seeking attitudes (Yousaf et al. 2015). A man's perception of how men should think and behave plays a significant role in shaping his attitudes and behaviors regarding access to mental health care. Social norms are critical. Complicating the issue, the authors noted that "men's ideals about masculinity may be exaggerated, which in turn may reduce their willingness to engage with psychological services. For example, if they believe that they should be stoical, but at the same time anticipate that health professionals will require them to be emotionally open and expressive" (Yousaf et al. 2015, 10).

Earlier work by Rickwood et al. (2005) analyzed data from 2,721 young people aged 14–24 years and reached similar conclusions, emphasizing the importance of tailoring messaging to meet young men's level of emotional competence. "Boys often do not recognise psychological distress for what it is, and if they do, they deliberately attempt to deny it and avoid exposing their distress to others," they wrote (24). "The social taboo of boys and men expressing their emotional needs may be slowly breaking down, but for the time being, boys still need to learn how to express their emotional needs in a way that is personally and culturally acceptable and empowering."

Medium matters. Although website- and video-based campaigns were the most common delivery modes, there was limited evidence of their effectiveness; in contrast, brief brochure-based campaigns were found to improve help-seeking outcomes (Duthie et al. 2024). Regarding content, campaigns featuring testimonials or narratives about mental health or suicide had a positive effect on help-seeking behaviors in general (Duthie et al. 2024). The use of storytelling helps men understand and engage. As Oschatz and colleagues observed, narratives may be perceived as less overtly influential and condescending compared to non-narrative health advocacy approaches (Oschatz et al. 2021). Similarly, Sagar-Ouriaghli et al.'s (2019) systematic review of men's help-seeking behaviors highlighted the importance of role models in normalizing mental health challenges. They wrote, "Using role models and supporting men to recognize and manage their symptoms were also of importance. This was helpful as role models often normalized the problems, offering reassurance that the difficulties were the result of everyday stressors. This made the problems more acceptable, enabling men to acknowledge their symptoms" (12).

A 2010 Australian study of 293 participants aged eighteen to twenty-five years old found young adult males were more likely to recommend seeking help from informal sources, such as friends, family, and websites. In contrast, females were more likely to recommend a combination of formal sources (e.g., counselors, general practitioners) and informal sources. The study utilized an online game designed to promote mental health help-seeking behaviors (Shandley et al. 2010). Notably, while the game was created with young men in mind, the researchers found that females benefited more from the intervention. The authors speculated that although the gaming element may have appealed to young men, the storyline resonated more strongly with female participants. This finding underscores the importance of designing interventions that align with male preferences—including narrative elements—to better engage young men in mental health care. As Shandley and colleagues noted, "These results support the evidence from existing studies identifying the Internet as a potentially critical way of tailoring and delivering mental health information and support to young males" (Shandley et al. 2010, 571).

Most importantly for our discussion, campaigns have the potential to drive immediate behavioral changes under the right conditions, even with brief exposure (Duthie et al. 2024). Notably, the majority of the studies examining help-seeking behaviors demonstrated a positive effect; in essence, efforts to guide men toward mental health care often succeeded. However, compared to women, men are significantly less likely to seek help for mental health challenges (Sagar-Ouriaghli et al. 2019). This disparity may stem from a lack of targeted messaging that resonates with men, leaving them feeling less invited or encouraged to seek care.

Ultimately, especially for young men, the most critical factor may not be the medium or the message but the messenger. In a study involving fourteen males aged sixteen to eighteen years old, researchers found that proximity and familiarity in key relationships were essential qualities when participants decided whom to seek support from for mental health issues (Burke et al. 2022). Feeling connected to the messenger was vital, making family members particularly effective sources of information about accessing care. Men's mental health outcomes are profoundly shaped by the social contexts and relationships they

Accessing mental health care depends on a critical trait or set of traits: the ability to seek and obtain that care. For those who need mental health support but do not receive it, the reasons are often deeply personal and varied. Among students, specific subgroups may have unique barriers to seeking help, necessitating tailored strategies to address their reluctance (Patte et al. 2024). Schools are frequently identified as key settings for the early identification of mental health problems and disorders. Yet, as Patte and colleagues observe, despite widespread initiatives to promote mental health awareness and reduce stigma, many students remain hesitant to seek support from school-based adults (Patte et al. 2024). Help-seeking reluctancy in school contexts remains common, particularly among students who may be most in need of support, according to the authors of a study of 70,794 students attending 136 Canadian secondary schools (Patte et al. 2024). Only about half of males and one-third of females in the study reported they would have no concerns seeking help for their mental health from an adult at school.

Doll and colleagues conducted a three-year community survey among some 307 people with mental health problems in Switzerland (Doll et al. 2021). Of their study group, only 22.5 percent of individuals with mental health problems sought help. The authors questioned whether "the health care system is offering enough low-threshold help-seeking opportunities for persons with emerging mental health problems, and how to design mental health care systems that are not associated with anticipated stigma, i.e., that identify features conveying anticipated stigma" (Doll et al. 2021, 9).

A primary obstacle to mental health care lies in what the authors describe as *functional impairments*—a concept that warrants closer attention due to its critical role in understanding barriers to treatment and its relative underrepresentation in discussions of mental health. Functional impairment refers to the real-life consequences of a mental health disorder, as outlined in a study on measuring functional impairment (Weiss et al. 2018). Often, the presenting issue that brings a patient to treatment stems from functional difficulties, such as trouble at school, struggle maintaining friendships, or job loss. These are the individual's functional impairments, which, for many who need but do not receive care, may also inhibit their ability to navigate the process of seeking treatment.

Such impairments are frequently exacerbated by the very mental health conditions the individual is seeking to address, creating a cycle where the illness obstructs access to its potential remedy. This dynamic is particularly troubling given the importance of early help-seeking behaviors, which are not only critical for preventing the progression of mental disorders but also essential for mitigating further impairments in functioning and quality of life (Campion et al. 2012). Understanding and addressing functional impairments is therefore vital to reducing barriers to care and improving outcomes for those with mental health challenges.

Michel et al.'s 2018 study of more than 2,500 individuals aged sixteen to forty in Switzerland revealed similar findings (Michel et al. 2018). Many participants recognized their mental health struggles and expressed a desire for help yet lacked the capacity to navigate the series of decisions and steps necessary to access care. This lack of action was often compounded by the mental health issues themselves, which created or exacerbated functional impairments. As a result, individuals frequently delayed seeking help until a crisis emerged. "Individuals commonly do not seek help until problems are severe enough to cause issues in occupational and psychosocial functioning," the authors noted, adding that this behavior significantly contributes to "the already immense costs of mental disorders" (Michel et al. 2021).

A Dutch study reached a similar conclusion, identifying "individual functioning" as the primary barrier to care among the thirty-two adolescents and young adults with depressive symptoms included in their research (Eigenhuis et al. 2021). These findings underscore the critical role of functional impairments in delaying help-seeking behavior, highlighting an urgent need for interventions that address these barriers.

Functional impairments present a significant and often unavoidable barrier to care for individuals with mental illness. However, the mental health care system has been slow to acknowledge and systematically evaluate the existence and impact of these impairments. Consider attention-deficit hyperactivity disorder (ADHD) as an example. Weiss et al. observe, "It is remarkable that despite multiple, specific, and serious functional impairments in ADHD, screening and evaluation of functional impairment has yet to become routine in clinic settings or in research" (Weiss et al. 2018). In insurance-based health care systems such as that of the United States, screening and assessment are essential steps in formally recognizing a condition, thereby initiating pathways to care. The absence of routine evaluation for functional impairments underscores a critical gap in both clinical practice and research.

It is deeply tragic when someone recognizes a need for help, knows help is available, yet lacks the functional capacity to access consistent care. Functional impairments often mediate the relationship between depressive symptoms and quality of life, with depressive mood serving as the trigger for these impairments (Zhou et al. 2022). In their study of 1,385 Chinese patients with major depressive disorder, Zhou and colleagues used various scales and questionnaires to demonstrate how depressed mood induces functional impairment, largely through a loss of interest in activities, hobbies, or work. This raises a critical question: how can someone who has lost the ability to care about themselves be expected to take the necessary steps to seek care? Framing the issue this way highlights the unrealistic expectation that the availability of help alone is sufficient. These individuals need more than just accessible resources; they require interventions that address their impaired ability to engage with care.

Fortunately, research demonstrates that effective treatments can address both depressive symptoms and functional impairments. For instance, patients treated with desvenlafaxine (50 or 100 milligrams per day) experienced significantly greater categorical improvements in functional impairment compared to those receiving a placebo (Soares et al. 2019). Additionally, improvements in Sheehan Disability Scale (SDS) subscale scores were found to be significant predictors of functional outcomes, according to the same study. This underscores the importance of targeted interventions that go beyond symptom relief to address the functional barriers that hinder access to care.

Symptoms, with very few exceptions, have a statistically significant impact on functioning (Tanner et al. 2019). Tanner and colleagues observed that "there was often high variability in the strength of the association between the various symptoms of a specific disorder and functional impairment." A deeper understanding of functional impairments provides critical insights into effectively treating mental health conditions. In the case of major depression, symptoms such as fatigue or loss of energy, difficulties with thinking or concentration, and depressed mood significantly interfere with the ability to seek care, experience joy, and maintain a fulfilling life. The authors noted, "Disability in major depression may be primarily driven by fatigue, mood, and cognitive impairments and less by sleeping problems, suicidality or appetite/weight changes" (Tanner et al. 2019, 7). While all functional impairments stemming from mental health conditions are detrimental, emerging evidence suggests that certain impairments are more likely to predict—and exacerbate—disability.

Trauma, PTSD, and complex trauma uniquely contribute to functional impairments, including difficulties in accessing care. To better understand these challenges, Jellestad et al. conducted a meta-analysis of thirty-four studies comprising 14,206 participants, examining the extent of functional impairments associated with PTSD (Jellestad et al. 2021). Their analysis revealed significant impairments across all functional domains except communication when comparing individuals with PTSD to those without. This suggests that while individuals with PTSD may face considerable challenges in functioning, including accessing care, their ability to communicate remains intact once they engage with support systems.

Similarly, Birkley et al. (2016) conducted a meta-analysis exploring the relationship between PTSD symptom clusters and relationship functioning. Their findings highlight that emotional numbing was associated with marital and parenting difficulties, as well as broader family and intimacy problems. Avoidance symptoms also contributed to challenges in family functioning and intimacy. These insights are particularly relevant given the intimate and trust-based nature of the therapist-patient relationship, emphasizing the need for therapeutic approaches that consider these relational barriers.

A study of nearly 14,000 California college students found that those experiencing serious psychological distress reported receiving information about mental health issues at lower rates than their peers without such distress (Sontag-Padilla et al. 2018). This raises the question of whether students with psychological distress might actually receive the same information as their peers, but their functional impairments prevent them from fully hearing, processing, or retaining the information provided. This possibility underscores the need for targeted strategies to ensure mental health information is accessible and impactful for students with heightened psychological vulnerabilities.

The *stigma* surrounding mental health struggles and seeking treatment continues to pose a formidable barrier, particularly for young populations (Villatoro et al. 2023). In the Healthy Minds Study, which surveyed 104,729 students across 196 colleges and universities, 41 percent of respondents agreed with the statement, "Most people would think less of someone who has received mental health treatment" (Eisenberg et al. 2023). Surprisingly, however, only 6 percent of respondents agreed with the statement, "I would think less of someone who has received mental health treatment." This discrepancy reveals the persistence of a phantom narrative of shame around seeking treatment, one that thrives despite being largely unsubstantiated, atleast in the context of study.

The enduring stigma around mental illness is further underscored by findings from a Swedish study on young adults' mental health help-seeking behaviors. The authors observed that "young people only talk to their closest friends about how they feel and it is still not perceived as acceptable to feel bad"

(Hellström and Beckman 2021, 9). Participants reported that individuals with mental illness are often labeled as lazy, attention-seeking, or strange, reinforcing harmful stereotypes. To foster better mental health outcomes, it is imperative to address the internalized negative perceptions surrounding mental illness and help-seeking that prevail among many young adults.

Labeling emerged as a significant predictor of self-reported help-seeking behaviors and recommendations in a school-based study conducted across fourteen schools in an urban/suburban district in Texas, involving hundreds of students as participants (Villatoro et al. 2023). The same study found that heightened awareness and proactive stigma-reduction efforts—such as understanding stigma and engaging in behaviors that treat and destigmatize mental illness—were associated with increased help-seeking in both formal and informal contexts. One proposed strategy to mitigate stigma's impact is peer advocacy, wherein individuals encourage their peers to seek help. As the authors note, "the stigma domains of labeling, stereotypes, and separation/discrimination do not always influence or interfere with help-seeking in the same way when the help-seeker is oneself versus a peer" (Villatoro et al. 2023, 11). This disparity suggests that while stigmas may be consciously rejected, they may persist subconsciously, subtly impeding self-directed help-seeking behaviors while being less influential in the context of supporting others.

Pimenta et al. (2022) reached a complementary conclusion in their qualitative study of 250 adolescents aged eleven to fifteen years old. Their findings emphasize the importance of equipping young people to respond constructively to a friend's disclosure of mental health challenges. Interventions and mental health awareness campaigns that target such responses could play a crucial role in addressing barriers to support-seeking early, ultimately fostering a more supportive and stigma-free environment.

The barrier effect of stigma can vary widely depending on the culture, population, and study mechanisms. For example, only 5 percent of male and female Canadian high schoolers have reluctance to get care due to worries about what others would think and potential embarrassment (Patte et al. 2024). Yet, adolescents consistently report concerns regarding others finding out about their mental health status (e.g., mental illness diagnosis) or decision to seek mental health services (e.g., resulting in a loss of status) (DeLuca 2018). The findings of these studies suggest young people are more likely to have positive attitudes and intentions toward seeking help when they: (1) expect confidentiality and trust following disclosure, (2) perceive the benefits of seeking help as outweighing the risks, and (3) associate disclosure with positive emotions.

A 2019 study of Canadian undergraduate students found that lower explicit stigma was associated with females, those with a history of mental illness diagnosis, and those who have had a close relationship with someone experiencing a mental illness (Sandhu et al. 2019). Major matters when it comes to stigma. Faculty of Social sciences students had significantly lower explicit stigma scores than engineering students.

Chen and colleagues examined eighteen contact-based educational programs aimed at reducing mental health stigma in Canadian high schools and found students were particularly concerned with peer reactions and the fear of being labeled as deviant (Chen et al. 2016). The success of these programs was largely attributed to the inclusion of speakers with lived experiences, who shared their personal stories. These stories were most impactful when delivered by individuals in recovery, offering students a hopeful vision of a better future. This aligns with a broader truth about young adults: across cultures and generations, few things are more distressing than being perceived as fundamentally flawed or different.

While mental health stigma remains a concern for some students, a possibly related trait, *hyper-self-dependence*, can also be a barrier to care. In one 70,000-student Canadian study, the authors found that "preferring to handle problems themselves" was the most frequently reported reason for reluctance to getting mental health care (Patte et al. 2024). Underlying this stated self-dependence "may be partly related to their concerns about *confidentiality* and skepticisms about the value of seeing help from school adults," according to the study's authors (Patte et al. 2024, 10). Promoting the efficacy of care and the privacy of treatment should also be on the mental health care promoter's agenda. Other studies affirm confidentiality as a barrier for some. A Swedish study of 2,358 males aged 15–17 years found that almost all respondents valued confidentiality regardless of their mental health, with 83 percent valuing an explanation of how secrecy functions in this medical setting (Haraldsson et al. 2022).

At a fundamental level, awareness of the existence of services, as well as an understanding of mental health issues and their potential solutions, is essential. A 2021 study of 2,036 university students in Bangladesh aimed to evaluate mental health knowledge and awareness. The study revealed that, although students demonstrated some awareness of mental health issues, their overall knowledge was notably limited. This lack of understanding hinders their ability to accurately identify mental health challenges and provide appropriate support (Siddique et al. 2022). While social media may increase students' awareness of mental health issues and familiarize them with a few specific conditions, this level of knowledge is insufficient to foster meaningful pathways to recovery.

Race plays a significant role in determining access to mental health care in the United States. Research indicates that Hispanics face greater financial barriers to accessing mental health services compared to non-Hispanics (Pabayo et al. 2021). The demand for mental health care among people of color continues to rise. Notably, American Indian/Alaska Native college students have experienced the most substantial increases in depression, anxiety, suicidal ideation, and other mental health concerns, alongside the most pronounced declines in overall well-being (Lipson et al. 2022). In 2016, approximately one-third of American Indian/Alaska Native students screened positive for depression, a rate comparable to other racial and ethnic groups. However, by the 2019 and 2020 academic years, this figure had climbed to half of the respondents in this group.

Financial status is a critical factor in determining whether individuals can access necessary care. A 2023 survey conducted by the California Health Care Foundation and the National Opinion Research Center at the University of Chicago polled a representative sample of 3,431 adults aged eighteen years and older living in California. The findings revealed that 74 percent of low-income individuals reported skipping or delaying mental health care in the past year due to cost (California Health Care Foundation 2024). The impact of rising living costs extends beyond low-income populations; over half of all Californians surveyed also admitted to forgoing or delaying mental health care because of financial constraints. Among low-income respondents who skipped care, 54 percent noted that their mental health condition worsened as a result.

Financial barriers to mental health care are not unique to California. A 2022 study of first-year Canadian university students identified the cost, availability, and effectiveness of services as the most significant obstacles to accessing mental health care (Samuel and Kamenetsky 2022). The authors offered practical recommendations for improving mental health support on college campuses, emphasizing the need to expand access. They suggested enhancing hours of operation, reducing wait times, addressing costs associated with missed or rescheduled appointments, and offering telehealth options to meet students' needs effectively (Samuel and Kamenetsky 2022).

Health illiteracy is another barrier to care cited in the literature, including in this 32-participant UK study (Eigenhuis et al. 2021). Young people experience unfamiliarity and insecurity with regard to issues related to mental health and help-seeking, as the authors of a Swedish-based meta-analysis of help-seeking behaviors of young people with mental health issues found (Westberg et al. 2022). "Young people in the analysed articles expressed unfamiliarity with both mental health problems and not recognizing oneself," they wrote (Westberg et al. 2022, 12). "Lack of knowledge was frequently described both with regard to communicating, distinguishing and assessing emotions but also regarding where and when to seek help, leading to a sense of insecurity." The longitudinal work of Bonabi and colleagues supports the notion that higher MHL predicts use of psychotherapy, as does having a positive attitude toward mental health care (Bonabi et al. 2016). When an individual is already equipped with knowledge about mental health disorders, it helps improve their recognition, management, and prevention of such disorders (Jorm 2012).

Availability of care is fundamental to receiving care. In late 2023, the California Health Care Foundation and NORC at the University of Chicago polled a random representative sample of 3,431 adults aged eighteen or older living in California. It can simply be difficult to obtain mental health care, apparently. "More than half of Californians who tried to make an appointment, meanwhile, say they have had trouble finding a mental health provider who takes their insurance—compared to only 14% who report difficulty finding providers who take their insurance for physical health care," noted the study's authors (California Health Care Foundation 2024). This, despite 81 percent of Californians thinking increasing access to mental health treatment should be an "extremely" or "very" important priority for state-level policymakers in 2024.

"Californians have strong views on the need to improve treatment options for people experiencing serious mental illness—and they are increasingly frustrated with their own personal access to mental health providers," said Kristof Stremikis, director of Market Analysis and Insight at the California Health Care Foundation (California Health Care Foundation 2024). "The high cost of care, meanwhile, is a perennial issue we've seen in poll after poll: This year's survey finds once again that rising health care costs are negatively impacting the lives of millions of Californians."

Adults in California with household incomes below $40,000 are the most likely to report poor mental health, with approximately one in ten describing their mental health this way, according to a 2023 poll conducted by the Public Policy Institute of California (Thomas 2023). The same survey found that a majority of Hispanic people in California rated their mental health as good, only fair, or poor, and only 21 percent were aware of the #988 national mental health hotline, which connects individuals to services such as the National Suicide Prevention Lifeline. Low income can have compounding negative effects on mental health. A study of nearly 2,500 households in the predominantly Hispanic Washington Heights neighborhood of Manhattan, New York, found that among individuals diagnosed with depression, those who faced financial barriers to accessing mental health services or counseling reported significantly higher levels of depressive symptoms (Pabayo et al. 2021).

Certain groups of young people face distinct barriers to seeking mental health support, particularly those in the foster care system. Young individuals in out-of-home care, along with their caregivers, are often disengaged from mental health help-seeking behaviors, as Powell and colleagues observed (Powell et al. 2021). The barriers to care for this population reflect a familiar set of challenges, including stigma, service inaccessibility, concerns about confidentiality, exclusion from decision-making processes, and a lack of clinician understanding of the unique circumstances faced by individuals in care.

What Facilitates Getting Care

The literature identifies several key mediators that facilitate access to mental health care. Research from Ritsumeikan Asia Pacific University in Japan offers a compelling synthesis of major factors influencing care-seeking among individuals experiencing suicidality. Notably, this study's sample was highly international, comprising 268 students—75 percent of whom were international and 25 percent Japanese—at a university hosting students from eighty-six countries. This diverse sample enhances the study's credibility and supports its argument for the universality of its findings. Using four different models, Nguyen and colleagues identified three fundamental conditions that facilitate care for individuals with suicidal ideation (Nguyen et al. 2021). They concluded that a sense of connectedness is essential for help-seeking behaviors that counteract suicide-related thoughts. However, they emphasized that connectedness alone is insufficient.

The road to care is paved with belonging, care information, and positive social norms toward care (Nguyen et al. 2021). Romeo and colleagues go so far as to recommend that schools require participation in curricular and co-curricular activities that are intentionally designed to promote belonging and well-being

(Romeo et al. 2024). Their study, which examined subjective well-being in 369 American college students, argues that universities should monitor the well-being of students as "well-being is at least as important as traditional learning outcomes" (Romeo et al. 2024, 15).

Bryant and colleagues' 2021 qualitative study of 304 UK higher education students (82 percent females) used self-reports to reveal help-seeking behaviors (Bryant et al. 2021). They found that *sense of and connection to place matters in getting care.* Commuter students were more likely to seek help from their off-campus educational support system compared to those living on campus, and queer students were more likely to engage with services off-campus. The findings show that student help-seeking behaviors were related to a sense of belonging and ethnicity, the authors wrote. As students' sense of belonging to their university increased, so did their help-seeking behavior. The authors of a Dutch study echoed this, saying, "adolescents' surroundings (school, family, and peers) appeared to play a critical role in the recognition of depressive symptoms and encouragement to seek help" (Eigenhuis et al. 2021). This sense of connection can be facilitated by adults in the young people's lives, offering an opportunity for connection and change (Jagosh et al. 2024).

A study conducted in Jordan examined the predictors of help-seeking behaviors for mental health services among university students. Given Jordan's cultural differences from the United States, these findings may hold particular relevance for foreign-born Muslim populations within our communities. The study highlights two critical factors influencing help-seeking: students must first perceive mental health care as a viable option and must also be able to recognize and acknowledge their own mental health challenges (Aldalaykeh et al. 2019). The researchers found that during periods of psychological stress, only 13.6 percent of students identified professional help as a potential resource. Furthermore, depression literacy levels were notably low, with 57.5 percent of students experiencing mild to moderate depression. Similarly, a Canadian study of individuals aged seventeen to twenty-nine reinforced the importance of health literacy in facilitating help-seeking behaviors. This study emphasized the role of factors such as symptom recognition, acting on symptoms, digital tools, Internet resources, and mental health awareness campaigns in promoting access to care (Stunden et al. 2020).

Aguirre Velasco and colleagues conducted a meta-analysis of ninety studies to identify barriers, facilitators, and interventions influencing help-seeking behaviors for mental health issues among adolescents. Their 2020 study focused on conditions such as depression, anxiety, suicidal ideation, emotional distress, and general mental illness symptoms, excluding other disorders like psychosis and anorexia. The analysis incorporated studies published in English, Spanish, and French, revealing that prior positive experiences with mental health services and strong MHL were the most significant facilitators of care (Aguirre Velasco et al. 2020). Building trust with gatekeepers is essential, as the MHL developed through these relationships can yield substantial benefits. For instance, young people with higher MHL are more likely to recommend seeking professional help and to believe in the effectiveness of suggested treatments (Wright et al. 2012).

Young people's attitudes toward their mental health significantly influence their responses to targeted messaging. A British study of eleven- and twelve-year-olds developed a continuum model to help mental health communicators tailor their approaches more effectively. At one end of the spectrum are adolescents who are "motivated and solution-focused," guided by the observations and actions of others. These individuals are more likely to seek help actively or share their difficulties with trusted people who might facilitate the help-seeking process. At the opposite end are adolescents who exhibit skepticism, unmet needs, or a preference for self-regulation. These individuals may express apathy or distrust toward seeking external help, opting instead to manage their challenges independently (O'Neill et al. 2023).

Negative affect, or experiencing a persistently negative mood, can serve as a predictor of help-seeking behavior among young adults. A recent study examining help-seeking tendencies among first-year Canadian university students found that negative emotions were associated with a greater willingness to acknowledge psychological challenges and an increased openness to considering professional psychological assistance (Samuel and Kamenetsky 2022). The authors suggest that overwhelming negative emotions may be harder to dismiss, prompting individuals to confront their mental health needs. Furthermore, when negative affect is coupled with access to trusted advisors or supportive individuals, the impact of stigma surrounding help-seeking is notably reduced.

An effective antidote to stigma, at least among international college students, may be increased exposure to mental illness, as visibility fosters understanding. A 2024 study of 132 international students across fourteen US colleges and universities found that greater contact with individuals experiencing mental illness was significantly associated with reduced mental health stigma in this population (Knettel et al. 2023). The study also revealed that identifying as woman and originating from a collectivist culture were linked to more positive attitudes toward help-seeking, while students from individualistic cultures exhibited more negative attitudes. Since collectivism and individualism are deeply ingrained cultural paradigms, addressing these frameworks may be key to improving attitudes toward mental health care. The authors suggest that "future research should seek to assess whether such individualistic attitudes that prevent help-seeking are malleable, in addition to exploration of interventions that highlight the value of collectivistic attitudes in facilitating help-seeking" (Knettel et al. 2023, 8).

The Trust Issue: Misinformation in Public Health Communication

Promoters of legitimate mental health resources face significant challenges in combating the pervasive spread of misinformation, particularly concerning health-related topics. Research shows that false health narratives can disseminate far more rapidly than verified information, undermining public health efforts and disease prevention strategies (Sommariva et al. 2018). For instance, a University of South Florida research team conducted a content analysis of Zika-related news stories shared on social media from February 2016 to January 2017. Their findings revealed that rumors were shared three times more frequently than verified stories. Popular falsehoods included claims that Zika was a conspiracy, posed minimal risk, or was somehow linked to pesticide use. The prevalence of such misinformation complicates the public's ability to discern factual information.

While the remedy to misinformation lies in the dissemination of accurate and credible information, too few individuals actively seek to verify what they encounter online. A 2022 study conducted in Bangladesh highlighted this issue, finding that nearly half of the respondents never attempted to independently verify rumors or facts about COVID-19 (Hossain and Haque 2023). This underscores the urgent need for improved health literacy and proactive public education to combat the damaging effects of misinformation.

Correcting misinformation, once it has spread, is a significant challenge, especially on social media platforms, which have been described as "a threat to public health by facilitating the spread of misinformation" (Walter et al. 2021). A meta-analysis conducted by researchers at Northwestern University examined 6,086 participants across various studies and found that misinformation shared by peers was more difficult to correct than misinformation originating from news organizations.

The study highlighted several factors that enhance the effectiveness of interventions to counter misinformation. Corrections were more successful when participants had a personal investment in the health topic, when misinformation was disseminated by news organizations rather than peers, and when corrections were provided by experts rather than non-experts. This underscores the idea that while "anyone can start a fire, it takes an expert to put it out."

A critical factor in receptiveness to correction is an individual's personal connection to the health issue in question. Walter and colleagues noted that "the more one cares about an issue, the more likely they are to continue to update their knowledge of an issue, particularly when a factual correction is offered" (Walter et al. 2020). This finding emphasizes the importance of fostering engagement and interest in health topics to combat the spread of misinformation effectively.

2

Young Adults and Mental Health

A Media-Mediated Crisis

It should have been a landmark media event. In May 2023, the US surgeon general, Dr. Vivek Murthy, a specialist in internal medicine and public health, issued "a call for urgent action" to, in part, "create safer and healthier online environments to protect children" (Centers for Disease Control and Prevention 2023).

The nation's doctor was telling us the online streets where our children play are not safe for them. He wanted "policymakers, technology companies, researchers, families, and young people alike to gain a better understanding of the full impact of social media use" (Centers for Disease Control and Prevention 2023).

The potential negative impacts of social media use on young people read like the potential side effects of an impossibly dangerous prescription medication: increased risks of suicidality (Jaycox et al. 2023), increased risks of anxiety and depression (Shannon et al. 2022), with body dysmorphia a far too likely outcome, especially for young women (Gupta et al. 2023), and a better than one-in-two chance they'll be bullied (Vogels 2022), all while increasing the access that traffickers have to them (United Nations Office on Drugs and Crime 2021).

Surgeon General Murthy repeated his plea for a warning label on social media platforms through an op-ed in the *New York Times*. "A surgeon general's warning label, which requires congressional action, would regularly remind parents and adolescents that social media has not been proved safe," he wrote (Murthy 2024). "Evidence from tobacco studies show that warning labels can increase awareness and change behavior. When asked if a warning from the surgeon general would prompt them to limit or monitor their children's social media use, 76% of people in one recent survey of Latino parents said yes."

This chapter will summarize recent literature about the relationship between media, mental health, and young adults. Special attention will be given to research that explores the impact of literacy levels and social media on mental health-related issues.

Mental Illness Issues Often Appear Early in Life

If people are going to experience a mental health disorder in their lifetimes, there's a good chance the first occurrence will be when they're young. About half of individuals experience the onset of their condition during adolescence, with the illness emerging by age fourteen in a third of cases (Solmi et al. 2022). The transition from childhood to adulthood is hard, with one's roles and body quickly evolving, along with expectations placed upon them (Byrne et al. 2007).

Mental illnesses are no different from physical illnesses in that early intervention is key. For mental illnesses, effective interventions, therapies, and coping mechanisms put the individual on a path to wellness and assist in avoiding negative patterns that entrench psychological issues as life issues.

Young Adult Mental Health Right Now

The COVID-19 global pandemic significantly impacted the mental health of young people, who remain disproportionately at risk for suicidal and self-harming behaviors, according to a brief released by the World Health Organization in 2022 (World Health Organization 2022). Data from the Centers for Disease Control and Prevention's (CDC) Youth Risk Behavior Survey (YRBS), part of the broader Youth Risk Behavior Surveillance System, highlight concerning trends. As the largest public health surveillance system in the United States monitoring health-related behaviors among high school students, the YRBS reports both progress and setbacks (Centers for Disease Control and Prevention n.d.).

In certain areas, young people appear to be demonstrating greater maturity and self-regulation. For instance, rates of risky sexual behavior and substance abuse—historically two major concerns for parents—have declined. However, the report also reveals alarming increases in poor mental health, suicidal ideation, and related behaviors across nearly all youth demographics. The authors emphasize the gravity of these findings: "The rates of experiencing bullying, sexual violence, poor mental health, and suicidal thoughts and behaviors indicate a need for urgent intervention." Particularly concerning are the experiences of female students and LGBTQ+ students, who face disproportionately high rates of violence, mental health challenges, and suicidal thoughts and behaviors (Centers for Disease Control and Prevention n.d.). Almost three in five girls experienced persistent feelings of sadness or hopelessness in the past year, and more than one in four seriously considered attempting suicide. Calling some of the findings "dire" might have been a euphemism.

The Healthy Minds Study, a collaborative effort among ten universities across the United States and Canada, surveyed over 500,000 college students aged eighteen years and older (Eisenberg et al. 2024). Led by Dr. Daniel Eisenberg, a prominent expert in mental health and well-being at the University of Michigan School of Public Health, the study aimed to assess the mental health needs of college students, evaluate the effectiveness of campus resources, and identify both risk and protective factors. The most recent report presents a sobering portrait of the mental health crisis facing young adults in higher education.

Forty-one percent of college students experience major or minor depression. Thirty-six percent have an anxiety disorder, as measured by their experiences over the previous two weeks. Forty-six percent report "lifetime diagnoses of mental disorders," although this survey polled only undergraduates and some graduate students. Twenty-nine percent have been on psychiatric medication in the past year. Fourteen percent of college students reported suicidal ideation, and the same percentage reported an eating disorder. Furthermore, 29 percent reported harming themselves in the past year, not with the intent to die, but simply to hurt themselves (Eisenberg et al. 2024).

Despite the constant and widespread opportunities for connection afforded by social media, 61 percent of respondents reported feeling left out either some of the time or often, with the same percentage indicating feelings of isolation. Moreover, only 38 percent of college students demonstrated positive mental health, as assessed by the Flourishing Scale, an 8-item measure evaluating self-perceived success in critical areas such as relationships, self-esteem, purpose, and optimism (Eisenberg et al. 2024).

The findings of the National College Health Assessment conducted by the American College Health Association provide a stark portrayal of mental health challenges among college students. The Spring 2024 survey included 103,639 undergraduate students from 154 institutions. Almost half of the respondents tested positive for loneliness, as measured by the University of California, Los Angeles (UCLA) Loneliness Scale (48.5 percent). About one-fifth (19.5 percent) reported experiencing serious psychological distress, based on the Kessler 6 (K6) Non-Specific Psychological Distress Scale. Alarmingly, 10.2 percent of students indicated they had intentionally self-harmed—by cutting, burning, bruising, or otherwise injuring themselves—within the past year, a figure that rises to 28.8 percent among transgender and gender non-conforming (trans/GNC) students. Additionally, over a quarter of students tested positive on the Suicide Behavior Questionnaire-Revised (SBQR; 25.9 percent), with trans/GNC students reporting at an alarming rate of 60.7 percent. Over a quarter of students (26.3 percent) rated their stress levels as high within the previous 30 days (American College Health Association 2024).

Students themselves report that mental health challenges significantly hinder their ability to learn and succeed academically. Among those experiencing anxiety, 47.8 percent state that it negatively impacts their academic performance. The figure rises to 55.9 percent for students with depression, 44.1 percent for those with PTSD, 65.3 percent for those with attention-deficit disorder (ADD) or ADHD, and 50.3 percent for those experiencing stress. These findings suggest that greater availability of and access to mental health care could enhance students' academic outcomes and overall success (American College Health Association 2024).

By several measures, college students have not fully recovered from the mental health challenges exacerbated by COVID-19. The Center for Collegiate Mental Health at Penn State's 2023 annual report indicates that while social anxiety, academic distress, eating concerns, and family distress all increased following the onset of the pandemic, only academic distress has shown signs of decline. Social anxiety, however, continues to demonstrate the most significant thirteen-year increase across their scales (Center for Collegiate Mental Health 2023). Family stress has also continued to rise, potentially influenced by post-Covid-19 cost-of-living pressures, which may be contributing to more young adults living with their parents for extended periods. College counselors report that anxiety remains the most common presenting concern, with relationship problems emerging as a prominent issue. Additionally, trauma has steadily increased as a concern since the 2014–15 academic year.

It would be hard to blame substance abuse for these issues, as only 23 percent of students said they'd used marijuana in the previous thirty days, 76 percent of students reported being drug-free, and more than half of students reported that they haven't drunk at all. Seventy-one percent of students reported having exercised at least an hour or two in the past month, so to some degree or another, our college students are moving (American College Health Association 2023).

Young adults were among the populations most significantly affected by the mental health challenges of the COVID-19 global pandemic. Ibarra-Mejia et al. (2023) conducted a survey of 456 college students at a Hispanic-serving institution in late 2020 to assess the prevalence and severity of stress, anxiety, depression, and substance use. Their findings revealed high rates of mental health issues, with prevalence rates of 53.1 percent for anxiety and 37.3 percent for depression—substantially higher than normative levels for this age group. Similarly, Czeisler et al. (2020) investigated mental health, substance use, and suicidal ideation during the pandemic across the United States. They reported that 25.5 percent of participants met criteria for an anxiety disorder, while 24.3 percent had a depressive disorder. Hispanic populations, such as those prevalent in Fresno, California, were disproportionately affected, with Hispanic participants reporting higher rates of anxiety (35.5 percent) and depressive disorder (31.3 percent). Additionally, 40.8 percent of Hispanic individuals experienced comorbid anxiety and depressive disorders, compared to 30.9 percent of all respondents (Czeisler et al. 2020).

Mental Health and Impact on Education

Research consistently demonstrates a positive relationship between mental health and academic achievement, as highlighted in a 2020 meta-analysis of thirteen independent studies focusing on adolescents (Bas 2020). The authors emphasize the critical importance of strong mental health for adolescents, noting its significant impact on academic performance and its long-term consequences for employment, income, and other life outcomes. They further underline the role of schools as key intervention points for addressing mental health needs, given the large number of young people they serve and the strong correlation between mental well-being and academic success. Supporting student mental health is not only beneficial for individuals but also aligns with schools' broader goals of fostering academic achievement.

It is intuitive that mental health disorders negatively impact learning, and research supports this. A 2022–3 Chinese study of 600 students found that stress, depression, and anxiety are statistically significant predictors of academic performance, with stress showing the strongest association (Zhang et al. 2024). "Mental health explains a significant percentage of the variation in students' academic performance," the authors noted (Zhang et al. 2024, 104351). A small study out of Brazil revealed that psychometric indicators of severe anxiety and severe functional impairment predicted students with lower learning performance (de Sá et al. 2023). Research by Eisenberg and colleagues suggested that depression is associated with lower grade point averages, and that co-occurring depression and anxiety can increase this association (Eisenberg et al. 2009). Depression has also been linked to dropping out of school (Eisenberg et al. 2009).

"I've got a student who, pretty much every day for the past three weeks, has emailed me to say, 'I can't even get out of bed today,'" remarked Jim Perez, an adjunct professor at Olive-Harvey College, a community college on Chicago's far south side, in an interview with *NEA Today* regarding the mental health crisis on college campuses (Flannery 2023). This sentiment is likely shared by thousands of professors across the country.

Research emerging from the COVID-19 global pandemic reinforces the connection between mental health and academic success. Tang and He's (2023) meta-analysis of the relationship between university students' anxiety and academic performance revealed a small-to-moderate negative correlation between anxiety and academic outcomes (Tang and He 2023). The authors highlighted difficulties with emotional regulation and suggested that negative emotions diminish students' functional capacities for learning and completing work. Notably, the analysis found that factors such as a country's development level, student type, or the nature of the anxiety did not significantly alter the impact. Students with anxiety, regardless of location or context, were likely to experience diminished academic performance as a result.

Another older but large longitudinal study by Eisenberg and their team landed on similar findings. Depression is a significant predictor of lower grade point average (GPA) and a higher probability of dropping out; co-occurring depression and anxiety are associated with lower GPAs, and symptoms of eating disorders are also associated with lower GPAs (Eisenberg et al. 2009). "This descriptive study suggests potentially large economic returns from programs to prevent and treat mental health problems among college students," they wrote, "and highlights the policy relevance of evaluating the impact of such programs on academic outcomes using randomized trials."

Even a brief social-belonging intervention can significantly improve students' progress in college, particularly for students from historically underrepresented groups, according to a large-scale study involving 26,911 students at twenty-two diverse institutions in the United States (Walton et al. 2023). These interventions have been shown to enhance retention and persistence among these populations. "Belonging concerns are primary for many students as they enter college," the authors noted, adding that "the history and reality of racism and social-class exclusion in higher education means that everyday challenges such as feeling excluded or having a hard time finding a lab partner can take on a racialized or social class–laden meaning for specific identity groups: 'People like me don't belong here.'" They emphasized that addressing these concerns early is critical, as such fixed, global attributions can become self-fulfilling (Walton et al. 2023, 380).

These findings are supported by the work of Murphy and colleagues, who conducted a randomized intervention study with over 1,000 first-year students at a Hispanic-serving university in the Midwest (Murphy et al. 2020). The intervention aimed to enhance students' sense of belonging and was found to significantly increase the likelihood that racial-ethnic minority and first-generation students would maintain continuous enrollment over the following two academic years compared to multiple control groups.

High school students report that mental health challenges often hinder their academic success. YouthTruth conducted a 2022–3 survey of over 500,000 high school students across the United States, revealing that 48 percent of respondents identified depression, stress, or anxiety as obstacles to their learning—an increase from 39 percent in spring 2020 (YouthTruth 2024).

> These sobering findings are a stark reminder that while COVID's acute phase is behind us, its effects on students remain . . . Other facets of the student experience, including mental health and access to adults from school to help, that worsened during the pandemic have still not recovered—and gaps between student groups persist. The trends presented here raise important questions and will require a dedicated response from educators, policymakers, and funders. (YouthTruth 2024, 10)

A study conducted in rural China examined the impact of screen time and outdoor time on a large sample of junior high school students (N = 20,375). On average, participants reported approximately one hour each of daily screen time and outdoor time. The study found that adolescents who spent two or more hours on screens were 3 percent more likely to exhibit higher levels of behavioral difficulties, with the authors noting that "excessive screen time was associated with worse mental health" (Wang et al. 2023). Conversely, outdoor time was linked to improved mental health outcomes. Students who did not spend time outdoors demonstrated lower prosocial scores, with rates falling between 6 percent and 8 percent compared to their peers who engaged in outdoor activities.

Mental Health in California

On average, Americans with serious mental illnesses have life expectancies that are twenty-five years shorter than those of the general population, largely due to untreated physical health conditions (Wiener 2023). In California, where the research in this book is set, approximately one-sixth of the population experiences some form of mental illness, and one in twenty-four lives with a mental illness so severe that it significantly impairs daily functioning. Alarmingly, suicides among adolescents aged fifteen to nineteen years increased by 63 percent between 2001 and 2017, underscoring the urgency of addressing mental health care gaps, particularly for young people.

Young adults report the poorest mental health among all demographics surveyed in the 2023 Public Policy Institute of California study on Californians' mental health. Nine percent of individuals aged 18–34 rated their mental health as "poor," compared to 3 percent of those aged 35–54 and just 1 percent of those aged 55 and older. Furthermore, 20 percent of younger adults described their mental health as "only fair," compared to 15 percent of those aged 35–54 and 9 percent of those aged fifty-five years and older (Thomas 2023). Collectively, these findings indicate nearly three in ten young adults in California may be experiencing significant mental health challenges or are at risk of doing so.

Many children in California face significant challenges. One in six California adults report experiencing at least four potentially traumatic adverse childhood experiences, including abuse, neglect, and domestic violence (Bhushan et al. 2020). In a 2017 meta-analysis of thirty-seven internationally focused studies, Hughes et al. examined the impact of multiple ACEs on health outcomes. Their findings indicate that experiencing four ACEs is moderately associated with an increased likelihood of smoking, heavy alcohol use, poor self-rated health, cancer, heart disease, and respiratory disease. Additionally, the authors identified strong associations between having four ACEs and sexual risk-taking, mental health challenges, and problematic alcohol use. The strongest associations were found with problematic drug use and both interpersonal and self-directed violence (Hughes et al. 2017).

ACEs significantly increase the likelihood of a child becoming involved in the criminal justice system, as one meta-analysis concluded (Astridge et al. 2023). Another meta-analysis demonstrated that having any ACEs at all can elevate the risk of depression, regardless of the number of adverse experiences endured (Tan and Mao 2023). Yet another study found that "adverse childhood experiences exposure can result in different functional and structural brain alterations in adults with MDD or chronic pain compared with those without adverse childhood experiences" (Antoniou et al. 2023, 729). Experiencing what is euphemistically referred to as a "rough childhood" exposes young adults to a cascade of risks that threaten health, wellness, functionality, and longevity. Notably, Californians aged 12–17 years old experience major depressive episodes at a slightly higher rate than the national average, with approximately 13 percent affected both statewide and nationwide (Wiener 2019).

Efforts in Fresno

In Fresno County, California, ambitious efforts are underway to raise awareness about available mental health services. The Fresno County Suicide Prevention Collaborative, comprising government agencies, community organizations, nonprofits, and community members, convenes regularly to share knowledge on suicide prevention and to assess and implement best practices (Fresno County Suicide Prevention Collaborative n.d.). The Collaborative offers regular meetings, training, and a website with valuable resources and scripts designed to support conversations with individuals at risk of suicide.

Suicides are on the decline in Fresno County, while still happening far too frequently by any humane standard. Suicides steadily decreased from 114 in 2018 to 90 in 2021 (ABC30 2022a). Of the ninety deaths in 2021, seventy-nine were males. Most were in the twenty-six to thirty-nine year age range, and many were White males. The Fresno County Department of Behavioral Health participated in the fifth annual multi-county suicide prevention summit in 2024 (County of Fresno Behavioral Health 2024). In 2021, the department launched its MENtal health campaign (County of Fresno Behavioral Health 2021), intended to reach male community members in need of help. The campaign to reduce the stigma around mental health includes videos of local people telling their stories (Fresno County Department of Behavioral Health n.d.).

A 2022 report by the Community Health System analyzed the health care needs of Fresno County and its neighboring, smaller counties—Madera, Kings, and Tulare (Community Health System 2022). Together, these counties encompass a population of 1,761,174, with 990,204 residing in Fresno County. The report identified mental health as the region's most urgent health need, ranking it as the number one behavioral health concern in all four counties, including Fresno. Following mental health, the next most pressing health issues for Fresno County were diabetes (chronic disease), substance use, and maternal and child health. These rankings are particularly striking in a region where 43–50 percent of adults have either prediabetes or Type 2 diabetes (ABC30 2022b), compounded by high rates of alcoholism (Anteola 2021), substance addiction (Fresno County Department of Public Health n.d.), and fatal overdoses involving fentanyl and methamphetamine (Fresno County Sheriff's Office 2023). To be listed as Fresno County's most pressing health concern is to stand out in a deeply competitive field of challenges.

The Community Health System report highlighted that youth aged seventeen years and under are the most likely to report mental health concerns, with rates more than five times higher than those aged sixty-five years and older (Community Health System 2022). Young adults aged 18–24 years old are the second most likely group to report mental health challenges. Among the region's residents, multiracial individuals reported the highest levels of psychological distress, with 20.1 percent experiencing significant symptoms. Furthermore, all four counties—Fresno, Madera, Kings, and Tulare—exceeded California's average for the percentage of adults experiencing frequent mental distress, defined as symptoms occurring fourteen or more days per month. Disproportionately affected populations included American Indian/Alaska Natives (26 percent) and Asians (26.1 percent), both of whom identified mental health as the region's most pressing concern.

Nearly one in five regional adults (18.9 percent) reported needing help for emotional, mental health, or alcohol- and drug-related issues in the year preceding the study (Community Health System 2022). Among those who sought help, 43.4 percent did not receive treatment. The Healthy Fresno County Community Dashboard offers a slightly more optimistic figure, reporting that 40.1 percent of adults requiring behavioral health care did not receive it (Healthy

Fresno County n.d.). However, this raises critical questions: why did so many fail to receive treatment? While the report does not address these reasons, one might speculate that barriers related to health, mental health stigma, or gaps in media literacy may have contributed to missed opportunities for connecting those in need with available care.

Over 20 percent of Fresno County adults have ever seriously considered suicide, according to the *Healthy Fresno County Community Dashboard*. An estimated 17.6 percent of adults are likely to have serious psychological distress. Childhood and young adulthood are critical times for diagnosing mental illnesses, as about 75 percent of serious mental illnesses first appear before the age of twenty-five years old (Kessler et al. 2007). Local resources lag behind the rest of California, according to the authors of the Community Health System report (Community Medical Centers n.d.).

Getting Care

Despite a growing percentage of adolescents in California reporting symptoms of depression in recent years, less than one-third have received treatment, according to *CalMatters*. The article highlights that many of these young people live in communities with insufficient mental health care options (Wiener 2019). "If you have a child or a teen in trouble, there are vast areas of the state where there is no appropriate help," said Carmela Coyle, CEO of the California Hospital Association, in an interview with *CalMatters*. Fresno, the largest city in the San Joaquin Valley, exemplifies this disparity, with fewer than sixteen psychologists per 100,000 residents. By comparison, the Bay Area has more than seventy psychologists per 100,000.

This lack of access often means individuals do not receive the help they need until they encounter the criminal justice system. "Far more people in California with mental illness are behind bars than in hospital beds," *CalMatters* reported. (Wiener 2019). "Over 30% of California prisoners currently receive treatment for a serious mental disorder."

An international meta-analysis of studies examining college students' use of mental health services found that approximately one-third of students access services during their time at university. Around one-fifth use outpatient services, while only 1–3 percent utilize residential services (Osborn et al. 2022). "Our findings suggest where there is greater availability of support there is greater use, as indicated by higher use being associated with services offering a range of treatments," the authors observed (Osborn et al. 2022, 29). However, they emphasized that effective messaging alone cannot bridge the gap where care is unavailable. The study concluded that "current services described in the literature are not meeting the needs of all students" (Osborn et al. 2022, 29).

Studies using both national and regional US samples have found that four-year university students report higher use of on-campus mental health services compared to community college students (Lipson et al. 2021), despite the higher prevalence of mental health problems among community college students (Sontag-Padilla et al. 2018). According to *CalMatters*, as of 2018, the California Community College (CCC) system had more than 7,000 students per counselor, while California State University—the system in which I teach—had more than 2,000 students per counselor (Weiner 2019). The University of California (UC) system, which includes prestigious campuses such as Berkeley, had about 1,100 students per counselor.

Mental health, often referred to as behavioral health, encompasses a variety of services provided by individuals with differing levels of training. In 2022, Dr. Janet Coffman from the Philip R. Lee Institute for Health Policy Studies at the UC, San Francisco, conducted an overview of California's behavioral health workforce (Coffman 2022). She identified three levels of behavioral health occupations: licensed professionals (including psychiatrists, psychologists, marriage and family therapists, and social workers), certified professionals (such as substance use disorder counselors), and unlicensed occupations (including community mental health workers, case managers, service coordinators, and social services/social work assistants). The Central Valley (where Fresno is located) has the lowest ratio of psychiatrists, licensed clinical professional counselors, and marriage and family therapists per 100,000 residents of any region in California, and the second-lowest number of psychologists by a narrow margin.

The Central Valley is 43.1 percent Hispanic (US Census Bureau n.d.), yet only 7 percent of California's clinical counseling psychologists are Spanish-speaking (Coffman 2022). As Coffman's report highlights, "The behavioral workforce does not reflect the racial/ethnic and linguistic diversity of the state's population, especially in professions that require a doctoral degree" (Coffman 2022, 24). For example, in 2020, only 13 percent of graduates from doctorate-level psychiatry programs were Latino, compared to 54 percent who were White.

There aren't enough mental health care workers in California, and the numbers are trending in the wrong direction. Dr. Coffman concluded that the number of graduates of educational programs will not be sufficient to replace retirees or meet the growing demand for behavioral health services. Two out of three respondents of the 2024 California Health Care Foundation Survey told pollsters improvement is needed in the treatment of people with serious mental illness, with 42 percent saying "significant" improvement is necessary (California Health Care Foundation 2024). Over 80 percent of Californians said it is important for state policymakers to focus on increasing access to mental health care in 2024.

Care on Campuses

The National College Health Assessment, conducted by the American College Health Association, provides a detailed snapshot of mental health care utilization on college campuses (American College Health Association 2024). The fall 2023 survey included 18,755 undergraduate students from thirty-eight schools. Among respondents, 32.6 percent reported receiving psychological or mental health services within the past twelve months. Trans/GNC students were the most likely to access care (60 percent), while cisgender men were the least likely (19.4 percent), with cisgender women falling in the middle (35.5 percent). Additionally, 16.6 percent of college students reported being prescribed medication for a mental health condition in the past year, with trans/GNC students again most likely to be prescribed medication (36.9 percent), followed by cisgender women (18 percent) and cisgender men (8.4 percent). Overall, 36.5 percent of students reported ever receiving counseling for a mental health condition.

Despite numerous barriers to care, a significant portion of college students are receiving mental health treatment, a topic explored further in the next section. According to the Healthy Minds Network, 36 percent of college students reported receiving mental health counseling or therapy in the past year, while 29 percent reported taking psychiatric medication during the same period (Healthy Minds Network 2023). It is worth noting an important demographic characteristic of the study: despite its large sample size, 54 percent of respondents identified as female, 41 percent as male, and 4 percent as transgender or non-binary.

"Counseling centers have seen extraordinary increases in demand over the past decade," observed Michael Gerard Mason, PhD, associate dean of African American Affairs at the University of Virginia (UVA) and a veteran college counselor, in an interview with the American Psychological Association (Abrams 2022). He added, "[At UVA], our counseling staff has almost tripled in size, but even if we continue hiring, I don't think we could ever staff our way out of this challenge."

College students today might be more frequently counseled and medicated than ever before. The Center for Collegiate Mental Health at Penn State published its most recent annual report in 2023, providing a comprehensive dataset from ninety-five college and university counseling centers (Center for Collegiate Mental Health 2023). The report examines 185,114 unique college students seeking mental health treatment and includes data from 4,817 clinicians. It is important to note that the findings are based on students who received mental health care, not the general student population. In other words, these students represent those who managed to access services, not the entirety of those struggling with mental health issues on campus.

The report highlights several concerning trends. Rates of prior counseling and psychotropic medication use have increased over the past year and are now at their highest levels since the data collection began in 2012. Moreover, a record number of students are arriving at campus counseling centers with a history of prior counseling or medication. Notably, 47 percent of students who initiated services reported experiencing trauma, another eleven-year high. The primary contributors to this increase were childhood emotional abuse and sexual violence.

The mental health care provided by campus health and wellness centers is typically short-term in nature. According to the Center for Collegiate Mental Health's findings, clients attended an average of 5.7 total appointments, with a median of 4 sessions and a range spanning from 1 to 135 sessions (Center for Collegiate Mental Health 2023). Students requiring longer-term care placed significant strain on the system; 20 percent of students averaged fifteen appointments each, but this group accounted for 56 percent of all attended appointments, consuming over half of the counseling resources. This data suggests these students received more comprehensive care, albeit at the expense of broader resource availability. Counseling services also appeared to be shaped more by academic calendars than by the therapeutic needs of students; the most common reason for counseling termination was the end of the academic term (42.6 percent).

One potential way to increase the capacity of campus counseling systems is by improving student attendance at scheduled counseling sessions. Of the

1,259,380 appointments recorded, 76 percent were marked as attended (Center for Collegiate Mental Health 2023). A particularly encouraging finding from the report is the speed with which students are able to access care. Approximately 35 percent of students had their first appointment of the year on the same day it was scheduled, and 81 percent were seen within five business days or seven calendar days.

While the majority of counseling appointments still take place in person (40 percent), video visits are a close second, comprising 29.3 percent of appointments. The remaining sessions occur through audio or text-based communication (Center for Collegiate Mental Health 2023). Most appointments last approximately one hour, with two-thirds of sessions adhering to this standard length. The data also reveal significant demographic trends in mental health care access. Women are more likely to utilize campus counseling services, accounting for 62 percent of those receiving care. Furthermore, 65 percent of those receiving care were assigned female at birth. Minority students are also accessing mental health services in substantial numbers, representing more than one-third of all campus counseling visits.

The 2023 Student Voice survey, conducted by *Inside Higher Ed* and College Pulse, gathered responses from a nationally representative sample of 3,000 undergraduates at 158 two- and four-year institutions. Among students who accessed campus counseling services, appointment availability emerged as both the most effective aspect of the services and the area most in need of improvement, highlighting significant disparities in students' experiences with accessing timely care (Flaherty 2023). Additionally, only two-thirds of students reported knowing where to turn on campus if they or a friend were experiencing a mental health crisis. "A lot of universities just don't have the infrastructure to support every single student's mental health in a therapeutic capacity," said Markie Pasternak, senior manager of education at Active Minds, in the *Inside Higher Ed* report (Flaherty 2023).

In December 2021, the Legislative Analyst's Office, the California Legislature's nonpartisan fiscal and policy advisor, released a report examining mental health services for college students. The report highlights encouraging news: all 10 UC system campuses, all 23 California State University (CSU) campuses, and at least 90 of the 116 CCC campuses provide student mental health services. However, the report also raises concerns about the limited scope of care. While campuses primarily offer short-term counseling in individual and, occasionally, group settings, effective mental health treatment often requires long-term solutions that go beyond these temporary measures. Such care is essential not only for students' immediate well-being but also for supporting their development as healthy, productive citizens (Legislative Analyst's Office 2021). The report also reveals disparities in service offerings across California's higher education systems, suggesting a kind of caste system among students. "Whereas UC campuses tend to offer the broadest array of services, including psychiatry services provided by medical doctors who are authorized to prescribe medications, CCC campuses typically offer the narrowest array of services," the Legislative Analyst's Office noted (Legislative Analyst's Office 2021).

In California, mental health services at colleges and universities are largely funded through mandatory student fees, which are charged to all students regardless of whether they use the services or the extent to which they do (Legislative Analyst's Office 2021). In the UC system, students pay a systemwide Student Services Fee of $1,128 per academic year, which supports a range of services, including mental health care. Additionally, six UC campuses charge supplemental fees of $85 to $549 per academic year to fund physical and mental health services. At CSU campuses, including Fresno State, where I teach, health services fees range from $150 to $740 per academic year. CCC are permitted under state law to charge health services fees of up to $44 per academic year, and most do so. Since 2017–8, the state has also contributed funding to support campus mental health care, with the majority of this funding directed to community colleges. In 2020–1, CSU reported spending $45 million systemwide on mental health services, $30 million of which was derived from campus fees.

The International Accreditation of Counseling Services recommends that campuses maintain a ratio of 1,000 to 1,500 students per mental health professional, commonly referred to as a "counselor" (International Accreditation of Counseling Services n.d.). As of fall 2020, the UC system met this recommendation with a systemwide ratio of 1,138 students per counselor. In contrast, the CSU system exceeded this range, with a systemwide ratio of 1,958 students per counselor (Legislative Analyst's Office 2021). The CCC system does not track this ratio. However, according to the Chancellor's Office, most community colleges employ only one to three mental health counselors, indicating significantly higher numbers of students per counselor compared to the UC and CSU systems.

In 2019–20, UC campuses collectively provided counseling services to approximately 34,000 students, representing 12 percent of total UC enrollment.

Additionally, psychiatry services were provided to about 6,400 students, or 2 percent of total UC enrollment (Legislative Analyst's Office 2021). The CCC system, which recently began collecting utilization data, reported that about 59,000 students—2 percent of total CCC enrollment—received any mental health services during the same year. It is important to note, however, that these figures do not represent the full scope of care received by California college students. Those with long-term mental health needs are often referred to off-campus providers, where they are expected to rely on their own insurance—and, in many cases, out-of-pocket funds—to cover the costs of treatment.

The California Budget and Policy Center published a report in 2019 that examined the mental health challenges and needs of California college students (Ramos-Yamamoto and Rose 2019). "Years of rising demand in mental health services among California college students have contributed to longer wait times and growing pressure to improve access to these services," the authors observed. "Before students can receive counseling, many must wait up to a few weeks for an available appointment. Additionally, many campuses have inadequate counseling infrastructure, with appointments taking place in non-discrete locations" (Ramos-Yamamoto and Rose 2019). The report highlights several at-risk groups, including undocumented students (Canizales 2019), veteran students (Richman 2017), and LGBTQ+ students (National Alliance on Mental Illness n.d.), who may face heightened risks for mental health challenges.

Undocumented students are of particular concern in Fresno County, where the Migration Policy Institute estimates there are approximately 77,000 undocumented residents (Migration Policy Institute n.d.). Among them, an estimated 10,000 are between the ages of sixteen and twenty-four. Despite these numbers, only 6 percent of undocumented individuals aged twenty-five years and older in Fresno County are estimated to have earned a college degree, reflecting significant barriers to higher education and long-term success.

Students from low socioeconomic backgrounds with limited social support face heightened risks, particularly given the increasing costs of tuition, housing, and books, as well as the prevalence of food insecurity, as noted by the California Budget and Policy Center (Ramos-Yamamoto and Rose 2019). At Fresno State, approximately 80 percent of enrolled students receive some form of financial aid, according to the Division of Student Affairs and Enrollment Management's 2023 report (Division of Student Affairs and Enrollment Management 2023). Additionally, over 60 percent of Fresno State students are Pell Grant eligible, meeting the university's definition of low-income status. These students arrive on campus already at risk—before they even encounter the additional pressures of classes and assignments.

The California Budget and Policy Center report highlighted innovative efforts to address student mental health needs, including CSU Fresno's *Let's Talk* program. This initiative "has allowed counselors to meet with students anonymously for 20-minute sessions in locations around campus, during which the counselor assesses the student's need" (Fresno State Student Health and Counseling Center n.d.). The report's conclusion was unequivocal: California college students require greater support, and their campuses need adequate resources to provide it. "Increased mental health funding should be directed to prevention and early intervention as well as direct services for students, considering that the demand for these services already exceeds the availability at many campuses across the state," the authors wrote. "Adequately funding these services can help mitigate the negative toll that mental health conditions can take and help students succeed academically" (Ramos-Yamamoto and Rose 2019).

Statistics about the care students receive may not fully capture the evolving strategies of campus counseling centers as they diversify their services. "Early on, it was just about more, more, more clinicians," said Carla McCowan, PhD, a counseling psychologist and director of the counseling center at the University of Illinois at Urbana-Champaign, in an interview with the American Psychological Association (Abrams 2022). "In the past few years, more centers are thinking creatively about how to meet the demand. Not every student needs individual therapy, but many need opportunities to increase their resilience, build new skills, and connect with one another."

Although the use of mental health services has approximately doubled over the past ten to fifteen years, levels of psychological distress among students continue to rise at a much faster rate, with significant inequities persisting. A 2023 report by the American Council on Education highlights these trends (Abelson et al. 2023). Students of color and low-income, first-generation students experience particularly high levels of unmet mental health needs (Lipson et al. 2018). Additionally, community college students face greater unmet mental health needs compared to their peers at four-year institutions (Lipson et al. 2021).

The capacity of college campus counselors—and mental health care workers in general—has its limits, and those limits appear to be under strain. Nationally, a full-time college counselor manages an average annual caseload of approximately 120 students, with some counseling centers reporting averages exceeding 300 students per counselor (Center for Collegiate Mental Health 2023).

Mental Health Services, Information, and the Growing Need for Support on California Campuses

A 2018 study published in the *Rand Health Quarterly* provides valuable insights relevant to this research. The study surveyed California college students in 2013 and 2014, posing two key questions: whether students knew where to seek mental health or supportive services on campus and whether they had received information from their colleges or universities about mental health issues. While the data is somewhat dated, the study's sample size is substantial and diverse, encompassing 13,968 students across twenty-six campuses statewide who completed both parts of this cross-sectional survey.

Notably, the study excluded transgender students from its analysis, explaining that "transgender individuals commonly experience unique mental health treatment issues distinct from lesbian, gay, bisexual, and queer (LGBTQ+) and other students" (Sontag-Padilla et al. 2018). Additionally, the researchers focused exclusively on campuses that received grants from the California Mental Health Services Authority to enhance prevention and early intervention activities for student mental health. These grants provided additional resources, enabling the campuses to make a concerted effort in addressing mental health needs.

According to the 2014 RAND survey, 56.6 percent of California college students reported knowing where to seek mental health or supportive services on their campuses (Sontag-Padilla et al. 2018). In terms of mental health-related information, students reported receiving such information in roughly equal measure from online and in-person sources. Specifically, students were most likely to report accessing information about student mental health issues from online platforms (e.g., Facebook, email, campus websites, Student Health 101), with rates ranging from 59 percent for relationship difficulties to 72 percent for alcohol and other drug use. Similarly, in-person training or on-campus presentations were common sources, with rates ranging from 58 percent for alcohol and other drug use to 68 percent for guidance on helping others in distress. Conversely, students were less likely to receive information from online training provided by their campuses, with rates ranging from 21 percent for depression and anxiety to 46 percent for alcohol and other drug use.

The RAND team recommended a human network approach to disseminating mental health information on California campuses. They proposed that "one approach to better reach individuals who are more likely to struggle with mental health problems could be partnering with campus organizations that may be more likely to address students with mental health needs" (Sontag-Padilla et al. 2018). Additionally, they suggested that "it also may be beneficial to focus dissemination efforts on a narrower range of mental health topics." However, the reality remains that marketing budgets for student mental health services are often very limited, and even the most substantial budgets have their limitations in reaching all students.

Young Adults, Teens, and Media Usage

Adolescents are spending nearly nine hours daily on digital media consumption when accounting for streaming, video games, and other screen-based activities, as reported by the *Common Sense Census* (Common Sense Media 2022). Adults also struggle with excessive device use. According to a 2022 Gallup poll surveying over 30,000 adults, the proportion of US adults acknowledging they use their smartphones "too much" has surged from 39 percent in 2015 to 58 percent in recent years (Saad 2022). Among eighteen to twenty-nine year olds, 81 percent admitted to spending excessive time on their smartphones when asked, "Trying to be as objective as possible, do you think you spend too much time using your smartphone, or not?" At the same time, half of Americans agree with the statement, "I can't imagine my life without my smartphone."

Americans have a complex relationship with their smartphones, particularly young adults, who seem unable to separate themselves from their devices. A striking 95 percent of young adults keep their phones nearby during waking hours, 92 percent keep them close while sleeping, and 86 percent check them immediately upon waking. As Gallup researchers observed, "Americans, it seems, are increasingly being outsmarted by their own phones" (Saad 2022). Rather than seeking ways to limit their reliance on smartphones, individuals are increasingly using them to perform essential tasks, further embedding these devices into their daily lives. According to the researchers, younger Americans are particularly vulnerable to the negative outcomes of excessive phone use, including addiction.

A 2023 Pew Research Center study surveyed 1,453 teens aged thirteen to seventeen, exploring their use of social media platforms. "Today's teens are navigating a digital landscape unlike the one experienced by their predecessors, particularly when it comes to the pervasive presence of social media," the authors noted (Vogels and Gelles-Watnick 2023). The findings revealed that 95 percent of teens reported having used YouTube, two-thirds had used TikTok, and roughly 60 percent had engaged with Instagram and Snapchat. Female teens were at least 10 percent more likely than their male counterparts to use TikTok, Instagram, and Snapchat. YouTube remains a dominant platform, with over three-quarters of teens using it daily, while more than half reported daily use of TikTok, Instagram, and Snapchat. Notably, approximately 20 percent of teens described their engagement with YouTube as "almost constant." Social media trends, however, can shift rapidly. For instance, Facebook usage among teens declined sharply, dropping from 71 percent in 2014–15 to just 32 percent in 2022 (Vogels and Gelles-Watnick 2023).

A 2023 Gallup poll surveying more than 1,500 adolescents revealed that over half of US teenagers (51 percent) spend at least four hours per day using various social media platforms, including YouTube, TikTok, Instagram, Facebook, and X/Twitter (Rothwell 2023b). On average, teens reported spending 4.8 hours daily across seven tested platforms. Social media use increases with age among teens, ranging from an average of 4.1 hours per day among thirteen year olds to 5.8 hours per day among seventeen year olds. Among the platforms, YouTube and TikTok emerged as the most popular.

Across the whole sample, boys spend 4.4 hours per day on social media, while girls spend 5.3 hours, but personality plays as much of a role as gender. (Rothwell 2023b). As part of the survey, called the Familial and Adolescent Health Survey, adolescents were also tested on personality traits. The authors found that one of the "big five" personality traits acted as a predictor of increased social media use: *conscientiousness,* which pertains to self-control and self-regulation. Those scoring in the bottom quartile in terms of conscientiousness spend an average of 1.2 hours more on social media per day than those who are highly conscientious.

This aligns with global patterns in mental health. A 2022 analysis published in *The Lancet Psychiatry* examined longitudinal data spanning 1990 to 2019, covering 204 countries and twelve specific mental disorders (GBD 2019 Mental Disorders Collaborators 2022). The study found a 48 percent rise in mental disorder diagnoses over the past two decades, increasing from approximately 654.8 million cases in 1990 to 970.1 million cases by 2019.

An overwhelming majority of school principals and vice principals identify smartphones and social media as key contributors to negative mental health and learning outcomes among students. In 2024, NBC surveyed 559 members of the National Association of Secondary School Principals and the National Association of Elementary School Principals (NBC New York Staff 2024).

When asked whether student mental health has worsened or if young people are simply more aware of long-standing developmental challenges, 92.29 percent of respondents stated that student mental health has indeed declined. Furthermore, 42 percent of respondents agreed with the statement, "I firmly believe smartphones and social media are major causes of deteriorating student mental health." Additionally, 69 percent reported that social media is "more likely to make students feel lonely and depressed than it is to make them feel accepted and happy." When asked which groups experience the most negative impacts of social media and phones—boys, girls, LGBTQ+ youth, or if such negative impacts are rare—79.17 percent indicated that girls are the most affected.

One frequently cited argument for allowing cell phones in schools is their potential utility during a mass shooting. However, principals and vice principals—those directly responsible for emergency responses in such scenarios—largely disagree. When asked, "Do smartphones make classrooms safer in the event of a mass shooting?" more than 80 percent responded, "No. During a catastrophe it is safer for students to stay off their phones and pay attention to instructions inside the school" (NBC New York Staff 2024).

The Critical Intersection of Young Adult Mental Health and Media

"Over the past 15 years, smartphone technology has fundamentally changed how children interact with the internet, coinciding with a decline in mental health among young people," stated the National Academies of Sciences, Engineering, and Medicine in December (2023). This observation was part of a comprehensive report offering policy recommendations to safeguard adolescent mental health (National Academies of Sciences, Engineering, and Medicine 2023). Supporting this point, the report highlights that "algorithms that generate content recommendations can either provide young people with valuable health information or expose them to unscientific treatments."

The report, chaired by Sandro Galea—then serving as the Robert A. Knox Professor and Dean of the Boston University School of Public Health—emphasizes adolescents' unique susceptibility to the negative effects of modern media. "The differences between an adolescent brain and an adult brain mean that teenagers can be uniquely affected by social media use," the authors noted (National Academies of Sciences, Engineering, and Medicine

2023). They further explained that "adolescents have less-developed controls for regulating emotions, heightened sensitivity to rewards, and are naturally inclined to seek independence and explore new identities during this critical stage of maturation."

About a third of American teens say social media has had a mostly negative effect on people their age, while 9 percent say this about social media's effect on themselves (Vogels and Gelles-Watnick 2023). This is an interesting example of a kind of Third Person Effect, the cognitive bias that leads us to believe that mass media messaging is more likely to negatively impact others than themselves (Tsay-Vogel 2015). As Tsay-Vogel explains, this perceptual bias in media influence has been argued to have behavioral consequences—including young adults' misperceiving the negative impacts of their own media and social media usage.

Adolescents who spend more time on social media compared to their peers tend to perceive themselves as less conscientious and are more likely to have parents who impose fewer restrictions on screen time—both factors associated with poor mental health outcomes (Rothwell 2023a). According to Gallup research, 41 percent of teens who use social media for five or more hours daily rate their mental health as poor or very poor, compared to only 23 percent of those who spend less than two hours per day online. Additionally, parents of heavy social media users are more likely to report that their teens frequently experience symptoms of depression and anxiety (Rothwell 2023a). In surveys of adolescents, respondents who heavily use social media are more likely to report anxiety and depression than those who use the apps less (Twenge et al. 2018).

The impact of social media on young adults is not entirely negative; amid the alarm bells, there are beacons of hope. "From a positive standpoint, I think we can't neglect in the conversation the elements of social media and connection that have a positive impact on mental health," said Michelle Lipkin, Executive Director of the National Association for Media Literacy Education (NAMLE), in a personal interview on July 2, 2024. She emphasized, "For a lot of young people who are marginalized in their own living communities—the ones they interact with in person every day—there's many young people out there that find that connection, their people, their community, online. And that is an incredible positive and has an incredible positive impact on mental health."

Young adults seeking connection with peers often feel compelled to do so through corporate information-exchange systems like media and social media platforms (Hardey and Atkinson 2019). Despite its drawbacks, social media can foster meaningful connections and support among adolescents. According to a 2023 Pew Research Center survey, the majority of teens report experiencing several positive outcomes from social media use: 80 percent feel more connected to their friends' lives, 71 percent appreciate having a space to showcase their creativity, 67 percent find people who can support them during difficult times, and 58 percent feel a greater sense of acceptance (Vogels and Gelles-Watnick 2023).

The Outsize Influence of Media on Young Women's Mental Health

Dr. Jonathan Haidt, professor of social psychology at New York University, describes the impact of social media on young people as "the great rewiring of childhood" (Haidt 2024). In his book, *The Anxious Generation: How the Great Rewiring of Childhood Is Causing an Epidemic of Mental Illness*, Haidt argues that the rise in anxiety and depression among young women directly correlates with the widespread adoption of smartphones. "All the way through 2010, even 2011, there's no sign of a problem—on some measures, things were actually getting a little bit better," he explains. "But it's nothing compared to what it is today . . . All of a sudden, the lines for girls go up like a hockey stick. It's not a subtle thing. There's an elbow. It's like somebody turned on a light switch in 2012" (Haidt 2024).

Haidt further points to hospital admissions for self-harm among girls, which mirror the sharp increases in depression rates seen globally. "Why did depression rates rise for girls faster than boys all over the developed world? Unless someone can find some hormone-disrupting chemical that was suddenly sprayed over northern Europe, the South Pacific, the US, and Canada around 2012, there is no alternative explanation other than the smartphone" (Haidt 2024).

Haidt also emphasizes that social media's effects extend beyond individual users, transforming social life as a whole. "Social media is very different because it transforms social life for everyone, even for those who don't use social media," he wrote. Abstaining is no simple solution: a girl who opts out of social media may find herself socially isolated if her peers are engrossed in these platforms for hours each day (Haidt 2023).

The link between social media and adolescent mental health outcomes is well-documented. According to a Gallup survey, teens who spend over five hours per day on social media are 60 percent more likely to report suicidal thoughts or engage in self-harm, 2.8 times more likely to hold negative body perceptions, and 30 percent more likely to report significant sadness compared to lighter users (Rothwell 2023a). While not all mental health challenges can be attributed directly to social media, the correlation is strong, particularly for heavy users.

A meta-analysis of twenty-six studies involving over 275,000 participants found "small but significant associations" between social media use and psychological well-being. Notably, the analysis identified a trade-off: increased social media use was linked to higher rates of depression and anxiety, though some improvements in social well-being were also observed (Hancock et al. 2022). However, such macro-level findings may obscure individual-level variability. Depending on personal disposition and contextual factors, social media's impact can be substantial for certain individuals, underscoring the need for families to critically assess its effects on their well-being.

Young women are particularly vulnerable to the negative effects of social media, especially when exposed to idealized appearances. Tamplin et al. (2018) demonstrated that such exposure significantly reduced body satisfaction among young women, though this effect was mitigated for those with higher levels of social media literacy. Media literacy education can thus play a crucial role in helping young adults harness social media's potential for inspiration while minimizing its harmful effects (Kross et al. 2021).

The nature of social media amplifies these challenges through selective and idealized presentations of reality. A *Wall Street Journal* investigation revealed, for example, that YouTube's recommendation algorithm promotes increasingly extreme and far-fetched content to maximize user engagement (Mickle 2021). Algorithms, as Pat Condo an expert in online information reliability, explains, are designed to keep users scrolling to drive ad revenue, often by presenting provocative and emotionally charged content. "It is down this rabbit hole where misinformation thrives," Condo writes (Condo 2023).

Social comparison remains a core mechanism through which social media influences mental health. While comparisons can inspire, they often provoke envy, contributing to negative self-identity outcomes (Schreurs et al. 2022). Adolescents are aware of peers struggling with both consuming and posting positively biased content, yet this awareness does not necessarily mitigate its effects (Schreurs et al. 2022).

Finally, parental involvement remains a critical factor in mediating the effects of social media. However, many parents face their own media literacy deficits, which can exacerbate the challenges of digital parenting. Children's greater digital fluency—referred to as "reverse socialization"—further complicates this dynamic (Benedetto and Ingrassia 2021). Szabó et al. (2024) found that while parents frequently express concerns about addiction, pornography, and online harassment, many lack the knowledge and confidence to address these issues effectively. This underscores the importance of schools and educators playing a more active role in supporting parents' involvement in digital education.

Do young women truly want to spend as much time as they do on social media? How much agency do they—or any of us—really have in this context? An experiment published in the *American Economic Review* found that nearly one-third (31 percent) of time spent on social media results from what researchers describe as "self-control problems" (Allcott et al. 2022). The authors argue that this behavior reflects "inattentiveness to habit formation and partial unawareness of self-control problems." If individuals are unaware of these issues, how can they be expected to address them? Furthermore, it is particularly significant that girls are more likely than boys to report difficulty in giving up social media, with 58 percent of girls expressing this sentiment compared to 49 percent of boys (Vogels and Gelles-Watnick 2023).

Parents as Mediators of Social Media's Impact on Their Children

Parents and educators ideally work together to address the challenges of digital education, yet the rapid pace of technological development and children's intuitive engagement with digital devices often make it difficult for both groups to participate effectively (Szabó et al. 2024). Research consistently shows that the strength of the parent-child relationship has a greater impact on adolescent mental health than social media habits. According to a 2023 Gallup survey, "When teens report having a strong, loving relationship with their parents or caretakers, their level of social media use no longer predicts mental health problems" (Rothwell 2023a).

Parental supervision and screen time restrictions also correlate with reduced social media use. Gallup data reveal that adolescents spend 1.8 fewer hours on social media apps when parents "strongly agree" that they restrict screen time, compared to those whose parents "strongly disagree" (Rothwell 2023b). Across all levels of social media use, mental health outcomes are significantly worse for teens with weak parental relationships than for those with strong ones. Notably, among teens with strong parental relationships, the comprehensive mental health index does not vary significantly between those using social media for five or more hours and those using it for fewer than two hours, suggesting that a strong parent-child bond acts as a mitigating factor (Rothwell 2023a).

Despite the clear benefits of parental involvement, only one in four parents of children aged three to nineteen strongly agree that they restrict screen time. While parental education level has a marginal impact—graduate degree holders are slightly more likely to enforce restrictions—political ideology plays a notable role. Forty-one percent of very conservative parents strongly agree that they restrict screen time, compared to 26 percent of conservative parents and just 23 percent of moderate, liberal, or very liberal parents. Conversely, very liberal parents are more than twice as likely as conservative or very conservative parents to strongly disagree with restricting screen time (Rothwell 2023b).

However, effectively monitoring and relating to children's media use can be difficult for parents due to their own media literacy deficits. Children often possess greater digital competency than their parents, (Benedetto and Ingrassia 2021). Moreover, many parents lack a model for media literacy education to follow (Szabó et al. 2024). In their meta-analysis of parental involvement in digital education, Szabó and colleagues found that much research focuses on parents as mediators. Across these studies, parents frequently expressed concerns about addiction, pornography, and online harassment, yet more than half also reported a lack of digital knowledge. This knowledge deficit was associated with increased parental anxiety, while well-educated parents were found to be better equipped to support their children's digital education. The researchers emphasize the need for teachers and schools to involve parents more actively in digital literacy initiatives.

In addition to unintentional negligence or media illiteracy, some parents directly harm their children's digital identity through "sharenting"—posting content about their children without their consent. Adolescents often find such posts embarrassing or damaging to their online identity (Verswijvel et al. 2019).

Ultimately, relationships between children and parents, as well as between individuals and social media, resist oversimplification. Factors such as personality, culture, and external influences significantly shape how children respond to media and social media. As the Institute for Family Studies argues, future research on youth mental health and social media must consider personality traits and parenting dynamics to better understand outcomes and avoid bias in comparative analyses (Rothwell 2023a).

3

The Media Literacy Movement

Can Media Literacy Heal?

"I believe it can," Michelle Ciulla Lipkin said in a personal interview conducted by the author on July 2, 2024. "It healed me."

On December 21, 1988, Lipkin learned through the media that her father had been one of the victims of Pan Am Flight 103, which had been bombed by terrorists over Scotland.

"We had nothing but what journalists could find out," said Lipkin, the executive director of NAMLE (The National Association of Media Literacy Education) at the time of this conversation. "We learned about the crash on TV. We learned that there were no survivors on TV. We learned it was a bomb on TV. Like, it was just us and the TV . . . you know?"

Lipkin was seventeen years old at the time, born in an era before media literacy had become widespread. Media coverage of the event was intense. There was conflicting information about the details of the crash and the perpetrators responsible. There was dissenting information about how the victims died and extensive reporting on the multi-country investigation. Headlines in the *New York Times* alone could make anyone's mind spin: "Call Libya's Bluff on a Pan Am 103 Trial" (Lowenstein 1997), "Pan Am 103: The German Connection" (Emerson and Duffy 1990), "Palestinian Radical Denies Link to Flight 103 Bombing" ("Palestinian Radical Denies Link to Flight 103 Bombing" 1990), and "Flight 103: A Solution Assembled From Fragments and Debris" (Johnston 1991). It was an incredible amount for a teenager to process in trying to better understand her father's death.

"Until I became someone that I can say has media literacy skills, I was really struggling to understand why everything was being portrayed the way it was," Lipkin said, reflecting on how the media often overlooked the victims and their families. "You don't always see the whole story when you're watching the news, and now it's obvious. But at that time, at 17, at 18, at 22, I didn't know I had no [skills for digesting media coverage]. It never occurred to me to ask questions."

Lipkin is passionate about helping young people develop a clearer understanding of the world and themselves through media literacy. “For me, media literacy education is completely intersected with healing from my dad’s death,” she said. “Like, they’re totally the same thing, because I had to learn to have a very intimate relationship with media in order to, like, process the death, respond to the death, continue to understand the death. It’s just been a very personal journey.”

Lipkin believes that misinformation spread by the media isn’t just a problem in political and social discourse. It also affects personal identity, such as with issues like body dysmorphia or feelings of isolation exacerbated by media messaging. Moreover, the media sometimes distorts stories of significant life events, as it did with Lipkin’s father. Media reports initially led her to believe that her father had died in a fiery crater. In reality, research and time revealed that he was found six miles away on a sheep farm.

There was solace in uncovering this truth. “I would say, absolutely media literacy can heal,” said Lipkin. “And, yes, I’m actually an example of it.”

While Lipkin’s testimony is deeply personal and offers a powerful lens into the human impact of media literacy, it is also consistent with the pedagogical principles laid out by NAMLE. The organization defines media literacy as the ability to access, analyze, evaluate, create, and act using all forms of communication, with a particular emphasis on inquiry-based learning. According to NAMLE, these principles “articulate a common ground around which media literacy educators and advocates can coalesce” and are “a first step in the development of clear, measurable outcomes and benchmarks for US schools” (National Association for Media Literacy Education 2007, 1). Rogow calls these principles an “invaluable guide for inquiry-based media literacy education in a digital world marked by media convergence and Web 2.0 capacity (i.e., the ability to interact and participate)” (2009, 72).

Though this chapter foregrounds a lived experience, the broader media literacy education movement is well-supported by empirical frameworks that shape how students critically engage with media in both academic and health contexts. NAMLE’s principles, in particular, have been explicitly operationalized in numerous peer-reviewed studies, especially in the *Journal of Media Literacy Education* and related scholarship (e.g., Hobbs 2021; Mihailidis and Thevenin 2013). Additional studies illustrate how media literacy competencies have been measured, applied, and considered in diverse contexts of application. Knaus (2022) used the core dimensions of media literacy to argue in favor of broadening the theoretical basis of media literacy education toward a more action-oriented approach. Literat et al. (2021) used media literacy principles as a jumping-off point to better understand how game-based learning can enhance digital and information literacies.

The existing literature maps nicely onto NAMLE's definition and provides a pathway for evaluating media literacy as both a cognitive and behavioral set of skills. Hobbs and Jensen (2009) encourage science—and by proxy, health—educators to create more authentic educational experiences by combining the vocabulary and learning experiences of media literacy and science. Media literacy is intertwined with education, but also politics, sociology, psychology, history, and communication (Yildiz Durak and Saritepeci 2019). All told, this existing body of research reinforces the argument that media literacy education can be rigorously taught and assessed, and these competencies can be meaningfully connected to real-world applications, such as navigating digital pathways to mental health care.

Media literacy helps us control our reality in essential ways—and so much more. In this chapter, I will define media literacy, explore the media literacy and media literacy law movements, and examine research that highlights how media literacy can serve as the foundation for addressing various societal challenges, including those related to health and mental health.

What Is Media Literacy? A Range of Definitions

The concept of media literacy, as initially developed by Renee Hobbs, founder of the Media Education Lab, refers to the ability to use, critically analyze, and create information content (Hobbs 1998). Hobbs later described media education in the United States as "a child with a thousand names" (Hobbs 1994, 453). Sonia Livingstone further defined media literacy as the ability to access, analyze, evaluate, and create messages across diverse contexts, emphasizing a skills-based approach (Livingstone 2004).

Expanding the conversation to digital environments, Eshet-Alkalai and Amichai-Hamburger (2004) defined digital literacy as comprising a wide range of complex skills—cognitive, motor, sociological, and emotional—necessary for effective use of digital environments. They identified five key digital skills:

1. Photo-visual skills (interpreting graphical instructions),

and internalize the nuanced social behaviors that are readily demonstrated in embodied interactions.

A key responsibility of social media literacy educators is to equip individuals with the skills needed to navigate the increasingly interconnected digital and physical realms effectively. Polanco-Levicán and Salvo-Garrido (2022) emphasize this point, stating, "Social media, by making possible and favoring social interactions, bring with them requirements for people to perform adequately on digital platforms, understanding that there is no separation between the digital plane and the physical plane; therefore, a mutual influence is produced that could affect people's experience by being exposed to the dangers on social media that worsen without the skills to deal with such situations."

Social media literacy remains an under-researched field, as highlighted in a systematic review of fifty-four articles on the topic by Manca et al. (2021). Drawing on a New Literacy Studies theoretical framework, the authors offer an insightful categorization of social media literacy skills. They distinguish between "those that are transversal across different social media (global skills), and those that pertain to a specific social media platform (local skills) . . . [as well as] practices that are decontextualized (literacy as something to be acquired), and those that are situated and context-dependent (literacy through participation)." This approach emphasizes the duality of social media literacy, encompassing both universal competencies and platform-specific, participatory practices.

The study highlights an important bias in social media literacy research: an emphasis on global social media skills, with minimal attention given to skill sets specific to individual platforms (Manca et al. 2021). Similarly, most of the identified skills pertain to "decontextualized practices, with very few studies emphasizing the importance of fostering situated social media practices." This raises critical questions about how this bias extends to media literacy and social media literacy pedagogy. If educators are concerned about the specific effects of platforms like TikTok or Instagram, should they not focus on teaching students how to use—and critically evaluate—those particular platforms? Likewise, if the concern is that students are disengaged from or manipulated by local media, should media literacy education not emphasize the skills needed to navigate and critically consume local media content?

Much of the serious media literacy-related research comes from abroad, as it does in many fields. Turkish researchers engaged in a thorough nine-step process to develop a scale to identify the levels of media users' media literacy skills (Eristi and Erdem 2017). After collating answers from 322 preservice teachers, they developed a scale that consists of forty-five items gathered under the four main factors of the ability to access, analyze, evaluate, and communicate. It's one of numerous scales that can be applied to young adults in our classrooms or the citizens in our communities to better help them understand their current personal media literacy levels.

There are both market-based and Marxist approaches to media literacy. According to Lewis and Jhally (1998), the primary goal of media literacy is to help individuals become sophisticated citizens, rather than merely sophisticated consumers. This perspective emphasizes not only the understanding of media production—especially the structures of media industries—but also the reception of media, which includes audience reception theories and research. As they assert, "Media literacy is, therefore, a way of extending democracy to the place where democracy is increasingly scripted and defined."

Media literacy, however, is a multifaceted concept. As such, media education in the United States often faces a tension between two competing goals: preparing students for the workforce and cultivating their ability to be more critical and engaged citizens within a democratic society (Chen 2007, 92). As Chen aptly notes, "In modern society, media intertwines with every aspect of human life." These many intersections represent diverse areas that could each serve as the focus of media literacy pedagogy.

History of the Media Literacy Movement

Early models of media literacy education, like many of today's, were based on an inoculation model. Imagine each media source as a syringe containing either harmful or beneficial content. If exposed to a particular media message, its values and ideas could "infect" the viewer. The inoculation model, therefore, trains individuals to identify both harmful and beneficial messages, encouraging them to selectively engage with only the positive content. This approach draws on Inoculation Theory (McGuire 1961), which proposed that attitudes could be fortified against persuasive influences in the same way the immune system protects against viral attacks (Compton et al. 2016).

The term "media literacy" was first used in 1986 (Friesem and Friesem 2019). According to Friesem and Friesem, the initial efforts to reach a consensus on its definition can be traced to a debate between Len Masterman and David Buckingham, published in *Screen* in 1986, during which Masterman introduced the term. This marked the beginning of efforts to bridge media scholarship and pedagogy—an endeavor that continues to evolve some 40 years later.

The concept of media literacy advanced significantly in 1992 when twenty-five media literacy scholars and educators gathered at the Aspen Institute for the National Leadership Conference on Media Literacy (Aufderheide 1993). During this conference, leaders formulated a definition of media literacy as the ability of a citizen to access, analyze, and produce information for specific purposes (Friesem and Friesem 2019). They also noted that the emphasis of media literacy training varies widely, encompassing areas such as informed citizenship, aesthetic appreciation and expression, social advocacy, self-esteem, and consumer competence (Aufderheide 1993).

The leaders there talked about "dramatic challenges in the current landscape," including a lack of a central mission and mandate, lack of infrastructure and legitimacy, a lack of knowledge of the right teacher training, and a lack of a way to evaluate student outcomes (Aufderheide 1993). The leaders called the field of media literacy "sorely under-appreciated in the United States."

In 1998, Hobbs outlined "The Seven Great Debates" in the Media Literacy Movement, framing them as critical questions that remain relevant today (Hobbs 1998):

1. Does media literacy protect children?
2. Does media literacy require student media production activities?
3. Should media literacy have a popular culture bias?
4. Should media literacy adopt a stronger ideological agenda, serving as a tool for education, social change, and political change?
5. Can media literacy ever reach large numbers of students in K–12 American schools?
6. Should media literacy initiatives be supported financially by media organizations?
7. Is media literacy best understood as merely a means to an end?

"The way we answer these questions will shape the future of media literacy," Hobbs wrote (1998), "and will determine whether the movement can capitalize on our nation's growing awareness that something has to change about our relationship and dependence on media culture." These questions remain vital to the ongoing development of the field.

As the field of media literacy has matured and evolved, it has been adapted to reach specific audiences and purposes. For example, Irving and colleagues developed a media literacy program for high school girls (Irving et al. 1998). In their intervention, female students who participated in the media literacy program reported less internalization of the thin beauty standard and lower perceived realism of media images, compared to seventeen female high school sophomores who did not take part in the program. The authors note that teaching girls and women to become more active, critical consumers of appearance-related media may help to prevent the internalization of societal beauty standards, the development of body dissatisfaction, and, ultimately, the development of disturbed eating practices.

The 2000s saw the emergence of textbooks addressing media literacy from various perspectives, including *Theory of Media Literacy: A Cognitive Approach* (2004), which highlighted the overwhelming presence of information in modern society: "We cannot physically avoid the glut of information that aggressively seeks our attention in our culture . . . Without a good understanding of the media, their messages, and the effects, people can develop misunderstandings and misperceptions about their world" (Potter 2004, 19). This insight remains strikingly relevant today.

Although the number of media literacy courses in the United States has grown significantly over the past generation, substantial gaps in efficacy remain. In 2024, the News Literacy Project conducted a study of 1,000 individuals aged thirteen to eighteen years old, finding that half of the teens surveyed did not recognize branded content as an advertisement (News Literacy Project 2024). Additionally, about 40 percent of teens failed to identify sponsored search results as paid advertising. The authors recommend the implementation of both media literacy standards and instruction, backed by high-quality professional development. They argue, "Policies that only focus on standards may not reach the classroom level in a meaningful way, and policies that only focus on instruction may not have enough clarity and guidance on what to teach" (News Literacy Project 2024, 88). "By requiring both media literacy standards and instruction, teachers will get the clarity and support they need to provide high-quality, nonpartisan news and media literacy instruction to their students."

The Media Literacy Law Movement and Its Pedagogy

True story: The legislative aspect of the media literacy movement was inspired, in part, by a website about Martin Luther King Jr. written by neo-Nazis.

Americans have the tools and knowledge needed to navigate the economy and digital world" (US Congress 2023). The bill "further highlights the importance of AI Literacy for national competitiveness . . . and highlights the importance of supporting AI literacy at every level of education, and requires annual reports to Congress on the state of this initiative," Forbes said (Talagala 2023). It was referred to the Subcommittee on Communications and Technology, where it ostensibly remains.

This leaves individual state lawmakers responsible for setting the priorities and direction for the public schools. According to the nonprofit Media Literacy Now's latest Media Literacy Policy Report, which outlines the status of media literacy education laws for K–12 schools in the United States, there is "significant progress of state-level policymakers as well as other organizations and key institutions and individuals to recognize an urgent need for media literacy education and to take action" (Media Literacy Now 2024, 4). As of 2024, nineteen state legislatures across the United States have taken formal action on K–12 media literacy or digital citizenship education. Eighteen governors have signed related bills into law, and one legislature has adopted two resolutions addressing the issue.

The laws and implementation look different from place to place. Connecticut placed its media literacy mandate in social studies and also allocated funding in support of the measure (Media Literacy Now 2024). New Mexico is requiring professional development. Virginia has an Internet safety law that Media Literacy Now classifies as media literacy education. There are at least nine states with media literacy-related legislation pending.

Some on the right have charged that media literacy laws are, in effect, an effort to indoctrinate young people with progressive ways of thinking, while others took up the cause of media literacy pedagogy in their fight *against* "wokeness." For example, in 2023, Florida's governor, Republican Ron DeSantis, signed into law a bill that requires students in grades six to twelve to learn how social media manipulates and distributes misinformation, as well as how to maintain personal security and identify cyberbullying, predatory behavior, and human trafficking on the Internet (Johnson 2024). Media literacy education can be many things to many people.

Delaware, as well, saw a media literacy education bill that was championed by an elected Republican. "The intent of the bill is to teach kids to think for themselves," said state Rep. Bryan Shupe (R-Milford), a Republican who cosponsored the legislation with state Sen. Sarah McBride (D-Wilmington), as quoted by *Delaware Public Media* (Nagengast 2023). "There may be some differences in curriculum from north to south . . . [but] If the districts take that to heart, it should be essentially the same across the state."

Here is a quick snapshot of two states on opposite ends of the country and how their media literacy legislation came to be.

New Jersey

New Jersey passed its media literacy law in November 2022. The bill was supported by a bipartisan colition, with all senators voting for the bll and unanimous passage in their house (New Jersey Legislature 2023). The bill broke new ground by being the first to mandate that school districts teach media literacy skills for students at every grade level from kindergarten to twelfth grade (Langreo 2022). The New Jersey bill directed the state's education department to hold public hearings about the new standards being created, giving the community an essential opportunity to be part of the process. New Jersey's state education department developed curriculum guidelines on media literacy with the help of a committee of certified school library media specialists and teachers across different subject areas and with the help of media literacy experts, as reported by *Education Week* (Langreo 2022). The bill fell short of requiring teacher training, though it had been discussed in earlier versions of the bill.

It's about "understanding the influence media has in our lives and the need to apply critical thinking to our involvement with media and to understand how to communicate using it," Sherri Hope Culver, a Temple University professor and the director of the university's Center for Media and Information Literacy, told *Education Week* (Langreo 2022).

Proponents did voice what could sound like progressive talking points to Education Week. "Here we are today where the very threats of our democracy are tied to mis- and disinformation," said Olga Polites, the leader of the New Jersey chapter of the nonprofit advocacy group Media Literacy Now (Langreo 2022).

In his press release announcing his signing of the bill, Governor Phil Murphy also talked about media literacy in grand democratic terms. "Our democracy remains under sustained attack through the proliferation of disinformation that is eroding the role of truth in our political and civic discourse," said Governor Murphy (Office of the Governor 2023). "It is our responsibility to ensure our nation's future leaders are equipped with the tools necessary to identify fact from fiction. I am proud to sign legislation that is critical to the success of New Jersey's students and essential to the preservation of our democracy."

In the same press release, State Senator Shirley Turner hit a more directly political note, saying, "This signing feels especially timely as we approach the two year anniversary of the January 6th attack on the US Capitol. It is incredibly important that our children are taught how to discern reliable sources and recognize false information" (Office of the Governor 2023).

The new state guidelines included seven directives, with many of them looking quite familiar to teachers of other courses like English and Civics/Social Studies: critical thinking and using information resources; research methods, including the difference between primary and secondary sources; the difference between facts, points of view, and opinions; and accessing peer-reviewed print and digital library resources.

Michael Testa, the Republican state senator and a lead sponsor of the new law, pushed back against this narrative. "By teaching kids to not blindly trust the information they receive through the news, social media, and other sources and giving them the tools to be skeptical, questioning, independent thinkers, we make it harder for them to be indoctrinated by anyone," he was quoted as saying in a release by the state senate (Testa 2023).

Strong support came from those that would implement the law: teachers. "At a time when misinformation and disinformation are eroding the foundations of that democracy, it is imperative that students have the tools they need to determine what information they can trust," said Sean Spiller, president of the New Jersey Education Association teachers union, in a statement quoted by Politico (Sitrin 2023).

California

The California bill—which passed unanimously—made history because, as the state with the largest number of public school students in America, every time they do something new it is history (National Center for Education Statistics 2024). Assembly Bill 873, which passed in November 2023, added media literacy to curriculum frameworks for English language arts, science, math, and history-social studies (California State Legislature 2023). Instead of a stand-alone class, the topic would be woven into existing classes and lessons throughout the school year (Jones 2023). California's bill did not include funding to train teachers, an advisory committee, input from librarians, surveys, or a way to monitor the law's effectiveness.

"We have a responsibility to teach the next generation to be more critical consumers of online content and more guarded against misinformation, propaganda, and conspiracy theories," said Democratic California State Assembly member Marc Berman, who introduced the bill, as quoted by *USA Today* (Martin 2023). "In addition, this instruction will help students to be more responsible digital citizens, more intentional about what they put online, and better understand online safety and privacy" (Martin 2023).

Those in education painted the stakes as high.

"The increase in Holocaust denial, climate change denial, conspiracy theories getting a foothold, and now AI . . . all this shows how important media literacy is for our democracy right now," Jennifer Ormsby, library services manager for the Los Angeles County Office of Education, told *CalMatters* (Jones 2023). "The 2016 election was a real eye-opener for everyone on the potential harms and dangers of fake news" (Jones 2023).

Again, there was some cynicism from leaders on the political right.

"A big problem with this new requirement is that today's news is as much about entertainment as information, particularly political entertainment," wrote Lee Ohanian, a senior fellow at the conservative-leaning Hoover Institution at Stanford University (Ohanian 2023). "Combine this with the fact that people like to hear what they want to hear, and you can see how these classes could devolve into 'CNN good; Fox News bad' in many California schools."

California has previously taken steps to equip its students with media literacy skills. Senate Bill 830, passed in 2018, aimed to "ensure that young adults are prepared with media literacy skills necessary to safely, responsibly, and critically consume and use social media and other forms of media" (California Department of Education n.d.). The legislation mandated the California Department of Education to provide educators with resources related to media literacy, including background information, project ideas, and lesson plans for K–12 teachers. However, the bill did not require mandatory media literacy education, highlighting the need for more recent legislative efforts to address this gap.

Merek Chang, who teaches science at Hacienda La Puente Unified east of Los Angeles, has been ahead of the curve teaching his students media literacy skills, inspired in part by misinformation related to COVID-19 his students believed from a tabloid. "The biggest impact, I've noticed, is that students feel like their voice matters," Chang told *Cal Matters* (Jones 2023). "The work isn't just for a grade. They feel like they're making a difference."

media skills. These gaps highlight the urgent need for comprehensive training in media literacy, especially in areas central to students' engagement with media in their daily lives.

McNelly and Harvey (2021) emphasize the critical need for enhanced training in media literacy, particularly in higher education settings and preservice teacher training programs. Their findings raise questions about whether current educators—both within their sample and in broader contexts—are adequately prepared to teach media literacy effectively. Addressing these shortcomings requires systemic support. As W. James Potter, a communications professor at the UC, Santa Barbara, argues, "Local districts must also devote financial resources to implementation. Otherwise, media literacy will begin to be regarded as a utopian ideal and disappear from the public agenda" (Johnson 2024).

Moreover, the delivery of media literacy instruction in the classroom inherently mirrors the values and perspectives of the instructor. Hobbs (2005, 75) observes that "educators have diverse and conflicting perspectives about the mass media. Most have a love-hate relationship with the mass media that is complex and multi-dimensional, and these attitudes and beliefs shape teachers' instructional practices in the classroom." This variability underscores the importance of equipping educators not only with knowledge but also with reflective tools to critically examine their own biases and attitudes toward media.

Part of what makes any ideal of uniform media literacy education so challenging is the fluid nature of media. What's relevant today is tomorrow's old news, over and over again. "That's why it's so hard," said Erin McNeill, then president of Media Literacy Now, to Sarah Schwartz in *Education Week* (Schwartz 2020). "The curriculum would have to constantly change to keep up."

The nonprofit and educational realms have made various efforts to help fill the gap by providing training and educational resources to teachers. Media Literacy Now's resource library contains just over 100 free resources for educators (Media Literacy Now n.d.). UCLA also has a useful library of free online resources (UCLA Library n.d.), as do the NAMLE (National Association for Media Literacy Education n.d.) and the Center for Media Literacy (Center for Media Literacy n.d.).

A December 2023 National Academies of Sciences, Engineering and Medicine report, Social Media and Adolescent Health, offered nearly a dozen recommendations for social media companies, Congress, the US Department of Education, and others to minimize the harm of social media use on adolescents' health while maximizing its benefits. Included among these were new curriculum standards and teacher training. "The Department of Education should draw attention to digital media literacy, and state boards of education should set curriculum standards for the topic," the authors suggested (National Academies of Sciences, Engineering, and Medicine 2023). "Teacher training should also emphasize digital media literacy, and the Council for the Accreditation of Educator Preparation should set requirements for student teachers and professional development for veteran teachers."

We can train educators to teach media literacy, but does it stick? As Share and Mamikonyan (2020) point out, English teachers play an essential role in helping students make sense of the boundless amounts of information they encounter, use, and shareand themselves disseminate. Share and Mamikonyan, both educators of educators, call for an expansion of what English teachers in America traditionally have taught, with an increased focus on what makes electronic communication unique and how to teach their students to think critically about all information.

Share and Mamikonyan (2020) utilized a unique subject set of their former students whom they taught critical media literacy practices during their education programs. They surveyed some 185 elementary and secondary in-service teachers to investigate whether former students applied critical media literacy instruction after graduation. Their results were optimistic, with the team concluding that critical media literacy "is not only possible for elementary and secondary English teachers to integrate into their instruction, but it is essential for their students who are immersed in this media culture 24/7," they wrote (Share and Mamikonyan 2020). "The first step in this process is to teach *with* media, using photography, music, social media, and a variety of information communication technologies" (Share and Mamikonyan 2020).

Media education is increasingly intertwined with social activism, yet scholars acknowledge significant ambiguity in its definition and a lack of a standardized approach (Turin and Friesem 2020). Social activism, however, encompasses a broad spectrum of often conflicting perspectives. For instance, one individual's activism might involve efforts to shut down a local coal mine to safeguard the environment, while a neighbor's activism could focus on preserving the mine—and the livelihoods it supports. These distinctions ultimately hinge on the values and interpretations of educators, teacher educators, and, ideally, the students themselves, who should be empowered to navigate and critically evaluate these complexities.

Media Literacy Works in a Lot of Different Ways

Media literacy serves as a versatile tool with applications across a wide range of desired outcomes. The existing literature demonstrates that media literacy can act as a powerful catalyst for positive individual change. Given the pervasive role of media in shaping our understanding of the world, any intervention aimed at behavior change may be incomplete without incorporating a media literacy component. The social norms conveyed through media profoundly influence consumption habits, self-perception, and behavioral patterns—including whether one accesses available mental health care.

On a basic universal level, media literacy has been shown to increase the critical thinking skills of young people (Feuerstein 1999). A study out of Israel found that media literacy education supports pupils' critical thinking about TV series and newspaper advertisements, and what's more, it also showed that there is a tendency to transfer such learning even some time after the program has ended. Those that might need the help the most—slower learners and the less affluent—benefited the most. According to the author, the program especially advanced the critical thinking abilities of pupils rated as low and medium school achievers and of those coming from a low-medium socioeconomic level. Higdon (2022) came to similar conclusions, saying that critical media literacy pedagogy strengthens students' analytical skills.

Media literacy programs specifically designed for women have been implemented globally, including in Peru through the *Media 4 Women* project. This initiative was primarily aimed at women and LGBTQ+ community leaders serving as students, teachers, and entrepreneurs (US Department of State 2021). The project focused on fostering a network of female leaders to promote responsible digital citizenship and empowering participants to combat misinformation. This included cultivating critical thinking skills to evaluate Peruvian media, influencers, and opinion leaders, as well as analyzing news and social networks in Peru. Similarly, courses such as Women, Girls & the Media at SUNY Empire State College encourage students to critically examine issues of authorship, production, and audience reception across various media forms—such as film, television, journalism, advertising, and digital media—to interrogate and challenge societal inequalities (SUNY Empire State College n.d.). By developing critical media literacy, individuals are better equipped to analyze and resist the distorted narratives and biases reflected in the media they consume.

Tugtekin et al. (2019) contend that media literacy significantly contributes to fostering democratic tendencies among university students, equipping them to critically evaluate media content and engage more effectively in democratic processes. Similarly, Ashley et al. (2017) found that media literacy enhances civic engagement by increasing students' knowledge of current events and their sense of internal political efficacy. Mihailidis and Thevenin (2017) describe media literacy as a core competency for participatory democracy, suggesting that media literacy educators play a pivotal role in empowering citizens to actively engage in democratic life. Another Turkish team validated this by finding a direct connection between media literacy and digital citizenship (Erdem et al. 2023).

Media literacy has demonstrated potential as a tool for combating domestic violence. Research shows that exposure to mainstream media is associated with more accepting attitudes toward relationship violence (Seabrook et al. 2018). The media content young people consume—and the critical lens through which they evaluate it—shapes their beliefs about whether it is acceptable for one partner to harm another. Lolita Moss, now an assistant professor at Tulane University School of Public Health & Tropical Medicine, conducted a scoping review of eight studies focusing on intimate partner violence (IPV) interventions targeting predominantly Black adolescent samples (Moss and Fedina 2022). These studies employed a critical media literacy framework, which Moss and Fedina, building on the work of Kellner and Share, define as "cultivating skills in analyzing media codes and conventions, abilities to criticize stereotypes, dominant values, ideologies, and competencies to interpret multiple meanings and messages generated by media text" (Kellner and Share 2005, 372).

The findings are compelling: educating young Black people about domestic violence significantly reduced their acceptance of violence in romantic relationships. Moss and Fedina advocate for integrating critical media literacy into IPV interventions for Black adolescents, emphasizing the importance of cultural tailoring and addressing power dynamics central to such violence. This approach underscores the adaptability and effectiveness of media literacy as a targeted strategy for addressing specific social challenges. For example, if a community seeks to reduce domestic violence, it can design a media literacy program centered on deconstructing harmful media messages and fostering healthier relationship norms. Similarly, if the goal is to encourage young people with mental health issues to seek help, a media literacy program could focus on reducing stigma and promoting positive representations of mental health care.

Media literacy, tailored to address the unique needs of a community, offers a powerful tool for driving social change.

Of course, media literacy education is also effective at helping people identify things like bias and news based on false information (Guess et al. 2020). Being social media literate has been shown to protect high school students from the artificiality and unrealistic nature of positively biased posts (Burnette et al. 2017). Media literacy programs have a significant positive effect on participants' knowledge, criticism, and awareness of the influence of media, as found by a large meta-analysis (Jeong et al. 2012). A Nigerian study found a wide range of ways that social media literacy skills "significantly moderate" the relationship between an individual and the social media they consume (Edegoh et al. 2022). When someone has lower social media literacy, they are more susceptible to questionable information sharing, status-seeking, the perception that "news finds me," and they are more likely to trust what they find on social media.

How Media Literacy Can Heal: Media Literacy-Centered Health/Behavior Interventions

Public health experts have long acknowledged the potential of media literacy to mitigate harmful health-related behaviors. Organizations like the American Academy of Pediatrics, the Centers for Disease Control and Prevention, and the US Office of National Drug Control Policy have advocated for the integration of media literacy into public health strategies to address these issues (Primack et al. 2006). Similarly, the Society of Health and Physical Educators emphasizes the significant influence of media on young people, stating that "media messages shape young people's perceptions—whether negative or positive—about body image, healthy eating, gender and racial stereotypes, self-esteem, substance abuse, healthy relationships, and other public health issues" (McNeill and Carter 2024). This underscores the role of media literacy as a critical tool in promoting healthier behaviors and attitudes.

"There's been a series of things that have really led us to double down on this idea that health education has to include media literacy interventions, because so much of the information that everyone gets about health and about nutrition and about mental health and about all of those things is coming from the media," said Michelle Lipkin, executive director of NAMLE, in a personal interview. "It seems really obvious to me, the intersection that you can't fully address mental health issues or health education issues without looking at media literacy interventions because of the influence media messages are having on all of us."

Lipkin believes media literacy interventions are critical for supporting the mental health of children, teens, and young adults.

"We're not asking the right questions (about social media and teen mental health), and therefore, we're not going to come up with solutions that are actually helpful for young people because so much of that kind of cultural conversation doesn't even mention education interventions," she said. "How are we going to actually support young people? It's a very complicated situation that deserves some complex solution building."

Media literacy and health literacy are mutually reinforcing concepts, each enhancing the effectiveness of the other in addressing the mental health needs of young people. Berkman et al. (2010) define health literacy as "the degree to which individuals can obtain, process, understand, and communicate about health-related information needed to make informed health decisions." Building on this perspective, Nutbeam (2008) broadens the scope, characterizing health literacy as "the development of skills and capacities intended to enable people to exert greater control over their health and the factors that shape health." Together, these definitions underscore the interplay between understanding information and fostering agency in health-related contexts.

The health promotion literature offers a distinctive perspective on media literacy, framing it as both a skill set and a behavioral intervention. A 2022 *American Journal of Health Promotion* article highlights that "media literacy skills are manifested through a two-step process that includes first becoming aware that it is important to assess a message source and then by establishing if the message requires fact checking" (Austin et al. 2022). The authors conceptualize media literacy as a tool to navigate what they describe as a toxic information environment, enabling individuals to critically filter prior experiences and knowledge. They further underscore its importance in health decision-making, spanning choices such as dietary habits, vaccination uptake, and accessing mental health care services.

In their 2023 policy report, Media Literacy Now defines digital wellness as "education addresses the physical and emotional health impacts of media use, with attention to helping develop the conscious, balanced use of media that aligns with an individuals' goals for their health and well-being" (Media Literacy Now 2023). They relied on the Harvard Medical School/Children's Hospital Digital Wellness Lab, which defined digital wellness as "an intentional state of physical, mental, and social health that occurs with mindful engagement with the digital and natural environment" (Harvard Medical School/Children's Hospital Digital Wellness Lab n.d.).

Let us now examine specific examples demonstrating the effectiveness of media literacy interventions in promoting healthier behaviors and outcomes.

Smoking and Drinking

Media literacy has long been a tool in smoking prevention, particularly among young people, by helping them critically assess the motives behind tobacco advertising. A notable 2001 study by Beltramini and Bridge (2001) involved 166 urban youth aged ten to fourteen years in a school-based educational intervention. Participants were encouraged to engage with questions such as, "Do tobacco advertisements tell us all the bad things that tobacco can do to our bodies?" and "Do tobacco advertisements want us to use tobacco?" The results were compelling: students in the intervention group demonstrated a significant increase in their understanding of the manipulative role of tobacco advertising. Furthermore, 24 percent of participants shifted from intending to smoke in the future to intending not to smoke, underscoring the potential of media literacy interventions to influence behavioral intentions.

Primack and colleagues (2006) developed a smoking media literacy scale for adolescents, demonstrating that smoking media literacy can be measured with excellent reliability. They argue that media literacy represents a promising tool for future tobacco control interventions, particularly given the limited success of traditional school-based smoking prevention programs in influencing clinically relevant smoking behaviors. This perspective aligns with research published in *The Lancet*, which links exposure to smoking in movies with adolescent smoking initiation (Dalton et al. 2003). Viewed through the lens of the TPB, these findings suggest that a person's behavior is shaped by their intention, which is influenced by attitudes toward the behavior and perceived social norms.

Media literacy interventions could play a pivotal role in this context by fostering more negative attitudes toward smoking and countering the perception—often perpetuated by media—that smoking is a normative behavior. The 2006 Primack study worked with a total of 1,211 high school students aged fourteen to eighteen in Pittsburgh, and the results were strong: those with higher media literacy were less likely to smoke, less susceptible to smoking, less likely to have positive attitudes toward smoking, and more likely to have antismoking norms.

Media literacy interventions have demonstrated significant effectiveness in discouraging alcohol use among young people. For example, a study by Goldberg et al. (2006) found that adolescents who participated in a media literacy intervention—particularly those who had previously consumed alcohol—developed a greater understanding of persuasive strategies, more critical attitudes toward alcohol advertisements and advertisers, and stronger intentions to abstain from drinking compared to their peers in the control group. Meta-analyses further support the efficacy of such interventions in reducing youth drinking. Jones et al. (2015) validated the positive impact of media literacy programs, emphasizing their potential as a preventive strategy. Additionally, Park et al. (2022) reported that higher levels of alcohol media literacy in children and adolescents were associated with more favorable drinking-related outcomes, including reduced positive alcohol expectancies, diminished intention to drink, and decreased risk of alcohol consumption. These findings underscore the value of media literacy as a crucial tool in alcohol prevention efforts.

Body Dissatisfaction

Authors of an English study that looked at how media literacy can prevent body dissatisfaction found that despite the increase in literacy-based interventions across the global north aimed at mitigating body dissatisfaction, media literacy is only part of the solution. "Many young people can offer rational critique and awareness that popular images are photoshopped, but this is not the same as producing capacity to move outside of entanglements of desire with these images," they wrote (Ni Shuilleabhain et al. 2021). Other researchers looking at school-based eating disorder interventions concluded that media literacy programs combined with an interactive, student-centered framework may potentially be a safe and effective way of reducing risk factors for eating disorders (Wade et al. 2003).

Media literacy interventions have proven effective in enhancing body satisfaction and addressing risk factors for eating disorders. A meta-analysis of school-based intervention programs involving 7,392 participants revealed that these interventions significantly increased body satisfaction while reducing perfectionism and thinness ideals (Kurz et al. 2022). Similarly, a pilot study demonstrated that media literacy programs reduced the internalization of appearance ideals and decreased body dissatisfaction, highlighting their impact on body image concerns (McLean et al. 2017).

Further research on an intervention targeting college women to address eating disorder risk factors, including bulimia, reported notable improvements in body image and a reduction in disordered eating behaviors (Szabo et al. 2012). Collectively, these findings underscore the potential of media literacy interventions to mitigate risk factors associated with bulimia and other eating disorders, supporting their role as a valuable tool in prevention and treatment strategies.

Intention to Get Vaccines

The COVID-19 global pandemic provided an urgent call to examine how media literacy can assist in health behavior interventions. A study led by an interdisciplinary team at Washington State University used a survey sample of over 2,000 to determine that media literacy and science media literacy skills aid health behavior adoption by contributing to knowledge gain and expectancies (Austin et al. 2021). A study also led by Washington State's Erica Austin found that "self-reported media literacy for news content had the strongest association with vaccine intention" (Austin et al. 2022).

When people think critically about information sources, they are more likely to think critically about content. Austin and his team conclude that media literacy campaigns that help people discern credible sources of health information could be a "crucial tool" for future vaccine promotion and other behavior change campaigns (Austin et al. 2022). From abroad, a Chinese study found that media literacy skills protected individuals from bad information about vaccines while strengthening positive information exposure (Xin et al. 2022).

As one COVID-19-related study emphasized, there are numerous other mitigating factors along with media literacy when predicting things like intention to take a vaccine, namely political leanings. Borah and their team found that liberals with higher media literacy for content held lower COVID-19 misperceptions, but this did not hold true for conservatives (Borah et al. 2022). Media literacy efficacy is trumped, in effect, by tribal political influence.

4

View from the Mental Health Care Provider and Promoter's Chair

Media as a Gateway to Their Care

To explore the role of media literacy in facilitating or hindering young adults in the greater Fresno area from accessing mental health care, I conducted interviews with twenty-one mental health care providers and promoters. These professionals represented diverse sectors, including county behavioral health offices, campus mental health care centers, nonprofits serving disadvantaged populations, and private practices (where many manage their own promotional activities).

Participants were recruited primarily through email solicitations to various agencies and individuals, with additional subjects identified through the snowball method based on participant recommendations. Recruitment emphasized diversity, and the majority of participants were non-White, with Hispanic individuals comprising the most represented background. The study was approved by Fresno State's Institutional Review Board, and all participants provided informed consent before participating. Interviews took place between June and December 2024.

The interviews followed a semi-structured format: participants were asked the same set of questions in a consistent order, with flexibility for follow-up questions to probe deeper into their insights and examples. All interviews were conducted via Zoom and recorded and transcribed using the Alice app. Confidentiality was prioritized by anonymizing all data during transcription and analysis.

This study focuses on responses to fourteen key questions, resulting in over 33,500 words of transcribed data. A critical content analysis was applied to identify recurring themes and validate findings within the interview transcripts. The data were analyzed iteratively to ensure reliability and coherence in the identified themes. The analysis was guided by the TPB, which emphasizes the roles of perceived social norms, attitudes, and perceived efficacy as critical precursors to behavior change—including the decision to access mental health care.

The questions posed in the studies that make up Chapters 4 and 5—which mirror each other—were informed by existing peer-reviewed literature related to online and offline mental health help-seeking, digital mental health interventions, and assessing media literacy competencies.

In their study outlining recommendations for assessing media literacy competency, Pereira and Moura (2022) said, "Quantitative methods can provide important and relevant indications of overall trends in media literacy competences and can give an extensive picture of the population's media literacy levels" (89). The researchers noted that, "All media literacy dimensions necessarily mobilize a set of competences which can be studied, but not through the same methods" (83). The media literacy competency we seek to better understand here is how young adults' media literacy skills and views impact their ability to *access* mental health care, and the questions are framed to reflect that. In their study of youth media literacy competencies—including the ability to access media—Pereira et al. (2015) asked direct questions about media usage, such as "Within the last year, did you . . . " (85). In this book, I also ask direct questions about whether different media were used to access available mental health care.

As one of the early pioneers of the media literacy as education movement said, "The measurement of media literacy competencies is a fast-moving target" (Hobbs 2017, 14). To that end, there are questions related to currently popular social media platforms like TikTok and Snapchat. As Hobbs (2017) also points out, "each approach to measuring media literacy competencies embodies core values in relation to a particular set of goals, contexts and situations" (1). Attempts by researchers to understand media literacies often include asking participants to self-evaluate competencies, including the work of Simons and their team, who asked subjects to respond to statements like, "I can use media devices in a technical sense," "I can evaluate media content taking into account various criteria (e.g., accuracy of information, comparison of information, appreciation of aesthetic aspects)," and "I am aware of my own media behavior" (Simons et al. 2017). The questions used in this study seek to illuminate the core value of better understanding how media and media literacy function in the situation of mental health care *access* for young adults, and are written as suc

Open-ended or semi-structured questions are a common way of better understanding mental health care-seeking. In a study looking to identify barriers to mental health help-seeking in young adults in Britain, researchers allowed for a wide birth of responses with questions like: "In your own words, please describe why you chose not to ask for help for your emotional or mental health needs, there is no right or wrong answer" (Salaheddin and Mason 2016). This fostered the revealing of both cultural and self-stigmatizing beliefs around mental health and help-seeking.

In a similar manner, when Rickwood and their team were attempting to better understand young people's help-seeking for mental health problems, they asked direct questions about recent experiences with mental health care, including, "Have you ever seen a mental health professional (e.g., school counsellor, counsellor, psychologist, psychiatrist) to get help for personal problems?" In their effort to better understand whom young people trust related to mental health issues, they prompted: "Below is a list of people who you might seek help or advice from if you were experiencing a personal or emotional problem. Tick any of these who you have gone to for advice or help in the past 2 weeks for a personal or emotional problem and briefly describe the type of problem you went to them about" (Rickwood et al. 2005). The studies in this book use both types of questions as a model for the interview approach with subjects.

TPB is one of the most prominent theories used in social and behavioral sciences, including research aspiring to better understand health and mental health seeking (Adams et al. 2022). Adams and team conducted a systematic analysis looking at adult mental health help-seeking through the TPB lens, noting that "mental health services are underutilized due to low rates of help-seeking, leaving unmet mental health needs," and "TPB has been applied to understand the help-seeking process and in the development of behavior change interventions" (Adams et al. 2022, 160). They found the theory to be robust and applicable in this setting, concluding that "attitudes and perceived behavioral control were significant predictors of intentions" (160).

An Australian team that investigated help-seeking for mental health problems among older adults with chronic disease found that the TPB model accounted for 69.7 percent of the variance in intentions to seek mental health assistance (Adams et al. 2021). Another research team that worked with young adults from San Francisco used TPB to understand mental health help-seeking among young adults with depression (Zorrilla et al. 2019). The questions in the Zorrilla study were also direct, including, "Do you know anyone, family member or close friend, who has ever met with a mental health professional?" (238). Their findings suggested that the variables of the TPB, especially attitudes, predicted help-seeking intention among a diverse group of young adults.

Bohon and their team's research roughly mirrored the same age group as my subjects (i.e., college students) with a similar purpose (i.e., predicting intention to seek mental health services) and also used TPB. Rather than asking participants questions, as I do here, participants were asked to respond to statements such as: "I am confident that if I wanted to, I could talk to a doctor about depression," and "Most people whose opinions that I value would not approve of me seeking mental health services for depression" (Bohon et al. 2016). They called the TPB model an "an excellent fit" that "revealed that more positive attitudes about care and higher perceived behavioral control directly predicted higher intention to seek mental health services" (Bohon et al. 2016, 593). Tomczyk and their team investigated TPB in help-seeking for a community sample of currently untreated depressive symptoms (Tomczyk et al. 2020). They too concluded that "the theory of planned behaviour (TPB) seems to be a tenable model to explain help-seeking for mental health problems and thus foster help-seeking" (758).

The studies in this book focus on two distinct subject sets: mental health care providers and promoters (Chapter 4) and young adults (Chapter 5), with the goal of illuminating how these two groups can better access each other through media. Researchers commonly interview various stakeholders in the same health care process to better understand the continuum holistically, including O'Reilly and their team. O'Reilly et al. (2019) conducted focus groups with adolescents, mental health practitioners, and educational professionals to uncover the potential of social media in promoting mental health in adolescents. Other studies looking at young adults and mental health care seeking only interviewed young adults, including the work of Liu and Zhang, who interviewed 18- to 25-year-old young adults (Liu and Zhang 2025). They found their data set to be robust enough to "reveal through in-depth qualitative analysis how marginalization shapes and constrains young adults' mental health care-seeking journeys" (2).

While the study provides valuable insights, it is not without limitations. The sample size, while sufficient for qualitative analysis, may not fully capture the breadth of perspectives on a broader scale. Additionally, the snowball sampling, though effective for accessing hard-to-reach populations, may have introduced some selection bias. Finally, the online format of the interviews, while convenient, may have influenced the dynamics of participant responses compared to in-person settings.

The full questionnaire is included in the appendix for reference. Young adults were defined as individuals between the ages of eighteen and twenty-five years. Media literacy skills were defined as including things like the ability to access, analyze, evaluate, create, and act using all forms of communication.

Do Young Adults Have the Media Literacy Skills to Access, Evaluate, and Act on Mental Health Care Options?

When asked whether young adults in their community possess the media literacy skills necessary to access available mental health care resources, our mental health promoter and provider respondents were divided: nine believed that young adults have the skills they need, eight believed they do not, and four provided mixed or uncertain answers. Many respondents cited social media as a tool that has increased access to information about mental health care options, as well as a generational decrease in stigma and improved media literacy skills. One respondent observed, "Practitioners and agencies are actively using these platforms to promote services and share helpful skills," with another adding that such skills are increasing "by the day."

Culture was identified as a significant factor influencing access to mental health care. Stigma remains pervasive in many communities of color, including Black, Indigenous, Hmong, and Hispanic populations, and serves as a barrier to seeking help. As one respondent explained, "For example, in the African American culture, there's still a strong association of mental health with 'crazy,' which blurs the ability to access care even if resources are available." Regarding the Hispanic community, another respondent noted, "Mental health is, like, not spoken of. It's kind of like a stigma. So it's nothing that they would really want to talk about." Additional barriers include basic literacy challenges, limited Internet access, and insufficient digital literacy skills, all of which hinder young adults' ability to connect with available resources.

When asked whether young adults have the skills to evaluate the quality of mental health resources available to them, participants expressed even less optimism. Two-thirds of respondents (14) believed that young adults lack the ability to evaluate the quality of mental health care options, with only two respondents affirming that they do and five offering mixed or uncertain answers. An overreliance on social media and superficial resources was frequently cited as a key reason for this deficit in discernment. As one participant noted, "I think a lot of them go on TikTok and they think like they're doing therapy by learning about it and stuff." Respondents also doubted whether young adults possessed the critical media literacy skills needed to distinguish high-quality care from highly advertised options. "The loudest, shiniest thing is the thing that gets the most attention," a local therapist remarked, adding, "I'm thinking of things like BetterHelp."

Multiple respondents highlighted the inherently complex nature of mental health care, which they noted is often misunderstood or inadequately addressed across society. One participant observed, "Do I really have the capacity to decipher what's going to work and what's not going to work? A lot of it is just them winging it." Stigma was also identified as a major barrier, leading not only to reduced care-seeking but also to a lack of open discussion about mental health in homes and social circles. As one mental health promoter explained, "I think that because their experience with a lot of these resources is so limited and for so many of these communities, mental health resources as a whole are not discussed. Especially if a member of the family or a friend is pursuing mental health resources, it's not something that they often discuss with each other. It's harder then to be able to compare and be able to tell, 'Oh, this is a worthwhile resource,' or, 'This is not really working for me,' because there's just not a lot to compare to."

This lack of MHL leaves many young adults without the foundational knowledge required to determine which type of care to seek. For example, respondents noted a widespread lack of understanding about the symptoms associated with treatable mental health conditions. "I don't think that the literacy is out there with the youth, nor with their parents, nor with the community," one participant stated. "It's one of the big challenges." Participants also pointed to gaps in education provided by the mental health care community regarding the various types of care available and when each might be appropriate along an individual's mental health journey.

When asked whether young adults have the ability to act on available mental health care resources, the professionals generally expressed confidence in their efficacy. Sixteen respondents believed that young adults can act on available mental health resources, while five indicated they cannot. Barriers such as stigma, the scarcity of care, and the need for additional support were commonly cited as challenges to taking action. As one respondent explained, "From what I've experienced and from what I've heard from our mental health team, which is a pretty small team, they often note that just kind of making someone aware of the resources isn't enough. A lot of times that isn't going to be followed through on, because of discomfort, because of a lack of understanding of how to access that information, etcetera."

The professionals generally agreed that young adults possess the necessary media-related skills, such as navigating online environments and texting, to act on mental health care options. However, personal motivation and comfort level play a crucial role. "I think it's just a matter of accountability and being willing to take that next step, which really only an individual is able to answer and act on," one therapist observed. Parents were identified as a key factor in empowering young adults with the skills and confidence to seek help. One participant emphasized, "As parents, we need to teach our children that it's okay to reach out, and I just don't believe that parents are sharing that information or they're not aware of the information that's out there for them. So making sure that the children understand that, I think, goes both ways."

The Many-Edged Sword That Is Social Media as a Tool in Delivering Mental Health Care Options

When asked whether they consider social media to be a reliable source of information about mental health care services, respondents offered highly mixed opinions. Seven participants answered affirmatively, six expressed skepticism, and eight provided nuanced responses such as "it depends." Social media was described as a vast and varied landscape where the reliability of information depends heavily on the source. As one respondent explained, "You know, it's as reliable as whatever the source is. I think what's hard with social media is, like, what we've been learning about the algorithms, right? You only get the information that you've clicked on before."

Several respondents highlighted the risks associated with young adults encountering harmful or misleading content on social media. One therapist expressed concern about the potential for exposure to damaging treatment practices: "There's also different types of therapists who advertise things that are not actually helpful or they're misleading people about what they can do. So sometimes I think about conversion therapy and how that's actually not really helpful, right. It's actually more harmful." Others worried that young adults are too quick to trust attractive links and too likely to believe the information presented without critical evaluation.

Respondents emphasized the importance of taking active steps to verify the credibility of information encountered on social media. "I would say take the extra steps to ensure you're digesting the right information," one participant advised. "Take the extra steps to pop open Google because you saw something on Twitter and look it up." They elaborated further:

> A lot of the times you could be scrolling TikTok and you're self-diagnosing yourself, but you're getting it from someone on TikTok that may or may not be an actual counselor or psychologist, and that could be a problem, right? Because you think that maybe, oh, well, maybe I do have ADHD or ADD, or maybe I do have depression or anxiety, but you're not actually seeking care. And so self-diagnosing can be extremely harmful because you're not getting the support that you need and you're not actually getting clinically diagnosed. And that's a very big difference between someone who's clinically diagnosed versus someone who's just wandering the world with no real answers.

Young adults' ability to evaluate social media content is further complicated by their varying levels of media literacy, health literacy, and exposure to personalized algorithms. One respondent noted that these algorithms can sometimes provide locally relevant resources: "I do think it is effective in some ways if people are really looking for local resources and kind of tapped into those, that [local quality] algorithm of what's happening around me, what groups are being offered, what events are available in the community." However, they cautioned that the broader picture of social media is skewed by commercial interests: "It's not a clear picture because it's who can throw the most money at it, you know what I mean, in terms of what they're getting access to. So it really depends on their ability to, like, sift through."

Regardless of whether respondents personally trusted social media as a source of mental health information, many acknowledged its potential as a tool for outreach. "Nowadays, I feel like social media has become such a huge platform as far as, like, advertising and as far as educating not only about resources that are available, but also about, you know, just mental health in general," one participant explained. Another respondent, an administrator of mental health programs, added, "We've got to embrace it and we've got to figure out then, okay, how do we take these platforms and use them to be able to deliver information? And it can be very powerful."

When asked whether there is a social media platform best positioned to reach young adults in the community, TikTok emerged as the most frequently mentioned, with fifteen respondents identifying it as the top platform. Instagram followed with nine mentions, while Facebook and Snapchat were identified by three and one respondent, respectively. One participant was unsure, and another simply responded, "no." TikTok's ubiquity on young adults' screens was cited as a key reason for its dominance. "I think a lot of people are getting their mental health information on TikTok," one respondent observed. Another elaborated, "I think Instagram and TikTok, in terms of a younger generation, are going to be what's in, because video-related content, specifically video content that they can digest within a minute or so, is crucial because that's just the information that they're interested in looking at."

Respondents emphasized the importance of platforms where young adults feel safe and free from stigma. As one participant suggested, "Some kind of a platform that you could go to to get information on your own in private that's not stigmatizing in any way, then I think that would be great, especially if it's kind of local oriented or regional oriented in the sense that the information that's provided is local." Some respondents expressed that Instagram might be better suited to provide legitimate information and foster connections between users and mental health care providers. "(Instagram) feels like it has more potential for people to actually connect with real people," one promoter noted. "It's actually faster. We've had people connect with us faster, too, on Instagram than even through email sometimes."

However, the global nature of social media accounts often complicates the pathway from information to actionable care. "I'll have a client say, 'I saw this TikTok about late diagnosis ADHD,' and you're like, 'Okay, well, let's just try to, like, sift through that.' And where are these people (providing the mental health information)? I don't know that it's like helping people access services because they're accessing information, but there's no bridge. (It's not clear) who's actually accessible to them, because often these people are, you know, all over the country or in other places," one respondent explained.

Ultimately, respondents acknowledged that the most effective platform today might not remain so in the future. Social media preferences among young adults evolve rapidly. "The challenge with that is it's constantly changing," one participant observed. "Let's go back 15 years ago, and there was, you know, MySpace, right? I'm really dating myself now. And then, you know, a few years after that came Facebook. And now we're finding that no young person is on Facebook. Those are all my age and older. And so then it was Instagram, but then it kind of migrated. Now it's all Snapchat and TikTok."

I asked mental health care providers and promoters to offer advice for social media platforms seeking to reach young adults with information about available mental health care options. Social media companies, often criticized for harming young adults, could instead be leveraged to provide help. What can they do to support mental health, and what might legislators mandate to curb the negative impact of social media while encouraging positive engagement?

Two key themes emerged: the importance of sharing authentic personal stories of mental health recovery and providing genuine, clear, and educational content about the therapeutic process. "Find someone that already used it, and knows how to access [care]," one respondent advised. "Show them step by step. Show them how to [access care]." Respondents favored a peer-centered approach to content creation. "Personal testimony from their peers," one participant suggested. "We have really found success with peer support and youth-driven projects. . . . I think having them get involved in creating the content is what makes it more appealing to them." Another added, "More, like, real-life stories of vulnerability and getting them into more of their heart space."

Practitioners also called for greater transparency about therapy, including what it entails, how to access it, and how long it takes to see meaningful change. "It's not a quick fix," one therapist emphasized. "It's a long building relationship, and I often say it's the weirdest relationship we enter in to. But really stressing that this is not a quick fix." Respondents noted the importance of fostering security and trust in young adults, many of whom have endured significant challenges. "On social media, students might be experiencing depression, anxiety, PTSD, or struggling with the fallout of sexual assault or sexual violence. They aren't really going to react to something because maybe they're feeling [traumatized]," one participant explained. "I think if we're able to put a face behind, you know, someone talking about mental health, that helps. There's a human aspect to it. Be human, be genuine."

Much of the advice was practical. Respondents stressed the need for up-to-date information, financial details about care, concise and engaging messaging, and connections to local resources. Two practitioners advocated for stricter controls on mental health-related content from untrustworthy or unreliable sources. An administrator of a large mental health care system urged social media companies to amplify reliable mental health content: "How do we reach larger groups? How do we reach thousands of people?" she wondered.

Advice to Mental Health Care Communicators: How Young Adults May Best Receive Information about Mental Health Care Options

This section aims to provide insights for those seeking to reach young adults with information about available mental health care services. Using responses from participants, the findings are presented within the framework of the TFB: social norms, efficacies, and attitudes.

Social Norms

Cultural expectations and peer influence play significant roles in either facilitating or inhibiting access to mental health care. Many young adults in Fresno are first- or second-generation Americans, navigating dual cultural identities. "They're trying to live between these two worlds of their parents and that old school world and then who they are here in America," one respondent explained. Machismo remains a barrier in certain populations. "With our Hispanic community, and in particular the Mexican population, many of the males do not want to seek counseling services because they've been raised to believe that that's a sign of weakness," another counselor noted. "The females will come in, but the males, it can be a little more challenging."

Trust is also pivotal in Fresno's culturally diverse community. As one counselor put it:

> There has to be this understanding that culture is huge for youth, especially in our community. In Fresno County, there's a very diverse culture, and one's community values are going to dictate the way that they pursue anything online. When you connect with these youth, you have to have an understanding of how these cultural values have dominated their lives. Especially being young, they haven't had a chance to really go out and define their cultural values for themselves. It's still very tight-knit, and a lot of these Spanish speakers, a lot of members in our Punjabi community, they're going to stay very close with their families.

Social media remains the dominant space where young adults prefer to receive information, primarily because it aligns with their habits and provides privacy. "It's where they already are," one participant said. In addition to online communities, young adults prefer messaging from peers or relatable individuals over authority figures. "Being able to speak to somebody as an equal, as a peer . . . rather than, 'I'm here to tell you what to do,'" one respondent shared. Trust in peers enhances the effectiveness of messaging, as another noted: "They want to know if it's essentially been vetted out, like, for the vibes and such." However, stigma remains a significant barrier, reinforcing the need for nonjudgmental and safe spaces.

Perceived Behavioral Control

Young adults are perceived as limited in their functional abilities to evaluate and act on mental health care options. Critical thinking skills, such as evaluating online mental health resources and discerning credible information, are underdeveloped. "I think they definitely need to have some sort of lessons, like introductions of how that would look [to get care]," one respondent said. "Like how to access that, like what the platform is, how to use the terms." Fast-paced digital habits exacerbate this challenge. "Kids are so quick, so everything's at such a fast pace. I think they don't take enough time to stop and analyze a lot of the work that they're given."

Follow-through is another area of concern. Young adults struggle with basic tasks like sending emails, making phone calls, or rescheduling appointments. Social and communication skills also need development. "They don't have the people skills that we grew up with, and they will need more guidance, modeling, and patience," one respondent said.

MHL is particularly low. "There's a lot of things missing in the schools, including mental wellness and mental health," one participant explained. "Mental health literacy is very, very shallow, very low in the communities . . . across all communities, not just at-risk Latino, Black, or Asian communities."

Generational trauma further inhibits efficacy. As one counselor observed, "This is a generation of people that have experienced a different level of trauma. COVID has exhausted them." This exhaustion serves as a functional barrier, complicating the numerous steps required to access mental health care.

Attitudes

Perceptions of the complexity of the mental health care system often deter young adults from seeking care. Many feel overwhelmed by the sheer number of options and lack confidence in determining what's appropriate for their needs.

"There needs to be more education to talk about mental illness and mental health stigma," one respondent said. "They hesitate to ask for mental health services, but once we explain it to them, then they're willing to accept the services."

The overload of information on platforms like TikTok often leads to self-diagnosis, undermining trust in professional care. "They need help, they need support," one subject emphasized. "They need to know there are other ways of managing the world."

However, respondents noted that young adults are becoming more open to mental health care. "They really want it," one provider stated. "They don't know how or where to look. We need to make ourselves more accessible." Positive messaging and education are needed to instill confidence in seeking care and understanding its long-term benefits.

Ultimately, respondents emphasized the importance of building trust and empathy. "Take time to listen, take time to ask them what they might be going through and how you can help them," one respondent said. Another added, "Try to be in their shoes to understand them. Build a trust because they're at the age where they might not trust anybody."

* * *

When asked at what grade level information about available mental health care resources should be presented to effectively reach young adults in our community, respondents indicated an average level just below fifth grade, with sixth grade being the most frequently suggested level. As one respondent noted, "Sixth grade, with pictures." Suggested reading levels ranged from kindergarten as the lowest to eleventh grade as the highest.

When asked which languages should be used to effectively reach young adults in the community, respondents consistently identified English, Spanish, Hmong, and Punjabi as the most important, followed by Vietnamese, Cambodian, Armenian, Tagalog, Laotian, and various Oaxacan dialects. Respondents emphasized the deep interconnection between language and cultural stigmas, noting that addressing mental health in a person's native language can help overcome these barriers. They highlighted the initial trust that is fostered when potential care seekers are communicated with in their own language, reinforcing the importance of culturally sensitive outreach.

Finally, I asked respondents how they believe young adults in their community would prefer to receive information about available mental health care services.

The options provided included video, podcast/audio, written form, virtual reality, or in-person interactions. Video emerged as the most popular choice, followed by in-person methods, with podcasts and audio formats receiving multiple mentions. Those advocating for face-to-face communication were particularly emphatic. "In person has the bigger impact," one respondent stated. "Face to face." Another noted that while social media facilitates broader outreach, it does not necessarily lead to service engagement. "In order to really get them, like, connected, I would say in person, because that's the experience that I got from people I work with," they explained.

Navigating Mental Health in the Digital World: A Media Literacy Approach

Finally, this section synthesizes the interview data to propose a framework for a media literacy curriculum aimed at equipping young adults to access, evaluate, and act on available mental health care options. The insights presented here are derived from responses to questions about which media literacy skills young adults in the community should possess to effectively navigate mental health resources.

Attitude Toward Understanding Therapy and Mental Health Resources, Including Setting Realistic Expectations

Young adults may misunderstand therapy or have unrealistic expectations of its process and outcomes. They often don't understand basic elements such as insurance, copays, and how prescriptions work.

They need to be taught that therapy is a long-term process and requires active effort to reshape perceptions. It's about helping them to "understand the process of therapy. The educational part of it," one counselor said. "Understanding that it's going to take a good amount of time before you actually start to see a difference. I think it'd be good for them to understand that, part of it is they're going to feel worse than feel better." This pushes back against a fantasy version of therapy presented on social media where someone walks into a room and then walks out healed that day. "Something that works for everyone else could be a complete disaster for you," another counselor shared. "So they need to just explore."

Respondents emphasized that the healing pathway is rarely linear. "In mental health, you could have days where you're like, yeah, I'm ready to tackle it," a subject said. "I don't care if I leave my counseling session crying like I want to get better. I want to work through these emotions. But then there's some days where you're like, this is the worst experience I've ever had."

Attitude Toward Building a Mental Health Vocabulary

Understanding key terms and concepts like "specialization" and "treatment approach" fosters a positive, informed view of therapy. Young adults need "to be able to articulate what they need." A mental health vocabulary facilitates this. "If you're going out into the world and you want to seek counseling or seek group counseling or go to a twelve step because of sobriety," a respondent said. "You need to do your fair share of research and making sure that you're going to feel the most supportive that you can."

A mental health vocabulary empowers an individual to look critically at potential care providers. "I think that what they need is to be able to look at the credentials of the practitioner and to know to some degree, who the practitioner is, what they would need to be able to find, maybe their theoretical orientation," a respondent said. "Meaning, like, how they practice, what theory they practice from."

A mental health vocabulary can also inoculate them from the self-diagnosing trend numerous respondents mentioned. "Everyone's talking about how they're neurodivergent or they have attachment disorder, and it's very convincing (what they see on TikTok)," one respondent said. "But people in that age bracket don't have the knowledge to actually evaluate a diagnosis." Knowing terminology lays the foundation for the steps to come.

Social Norms and Helping Them Understand Cultural Influences

Cultural factors, family norms, peer group expectations, and media portrayals significantly impact young adults' views on mental health care. They need help understanding this. "Mental health is, like, not spoken of," said one promoter. "It's kind of like a stigma. So it's nothing that they would really want to talk about. So that's, like, another thing that plays a factor, the culture, how they perceive mental health." Or, as another said: "I think it depends on what their cultural aspects are and what the stigma is in their culture. So I can speak for the African American culture. I still, as someone who's been in the field for 15 plus years, get crap from people of like, 'So you're crazy or you deal with crazy people' because they have associated mental health with, like, loss of sanity."

Perceived Behavioral Control and Foundational Digital Skills

Basic abilities like navigating websites, using search engines effectively, or exploring apps are crucial for accessing resources. "There's the assumption that, Oh, they're kids, they've had an iPad in their hands since they were babies," one respondent said, "But a lot of them haven't. They just didn't have the money for these kinds of tools. They've never even used this. Their parents don't even know how to do email. And then we're like, 'Oh, you can't use Google. Like, figure it out.' And that's really where I think it needs to start. I think there needs to be more building block kinds of skills."

Self-regulation might not be traditionally thought of as a digital skill, but it takes patience to navigate complicated digital systems. "We're all going to get frustrated," one respondent said. "So, you know, teach me. Teach me what the way looks like. Teach me, you know, the lay of the land." This self-regulation is also the key to being able to ask questions, subjects said. "Being patient enough to slow down and read everything and understand everything is a media literacy skill itself," another respondent said.

"To feel is to heal," said one mental health provider. "You can't know that you're triggered if you don't allow yourself to feel it. Like, you have to feel that in order to be like, 'Oh, I'm getting triggered again in this moment. This is how I felt, just, like, in the therapist's office. Like, my heart was beating really fast, my stomach was, like, in knots.' And to be able to understand that and, like, then connected to when you're outside."

Perceived Behavioral Control and Practical Communication Skills

Skills such as making phone calls, writing professional emails, accessing Zoom, and completing forms are necessary for engaging with providers. "This generation of young adults is facing more challenges maybe than those in the past in terms of what's it like to make a phone call," one respondent said. "A lot of them don't have a familiarity with Zoom or video conferencing," another said. "And that's a big thing. Still, for a lot of local therapists here, they're still doing a lot of telehealth appointments. And so that, I think, limits our community even more because we're not providing the basic understanding of how to access that."

Perceived Behavioral Control and Critical Thinking and Evaluation of Sources

The ability to assess the credibility of mental health resources enables informed decision-making. In this case, that can mean, "possibly using insurance websites that have lists of providers that use, that take their insurance, being able to filter certain requirements or certain preferences that they may have," as one respondent put it.

Perceived Behavioral Control and Confidence in Taking Action

Many young adults need support to overcome fear of judgment, anxiety about seeking help, or unfamiliarity with the process. "For me, it's searching for the person that you feel is going to support you best," one counselor said. "They have a voice in that." They also need to have confidence to be open with their potential caregivers and caregiving system. "It's okay to not feel okay, but they need to express that," one respondent said. "They need to be very transparent. I know this sounds really basic, but the information that I hear from our therapist is that, let's say, for example, a student is depressed, but it doesn't come out until many, many, many sessions down the road that they are also abusing drugs, you know, smoking marijuana on a regular basis. That can be a problem when it comes to trying to seek mental health support. So I think that transparency with their therapist and really advocating on their own behalf."

* * *

Now, it's time to hear directly from the young adults themselves.

5

Meeting Young Adults in the Media Landscape Where They Want to Be Met

The responses from mental health care practitioners and promoters provided invaluable insights that should inform media literacy education and mental health care promotion campaigns. However, this study does not merely address young adults—it engages with them directly. Most importantly, it prioritizes listening to their perspectives. In this section, we present findings from interviews with thirty young adults (ages 18–25 years) residing in the greater Fresno metropolitan area. These participants shared their views on trusted media sources, preferred methods for receiving information about mental health care, and the cultural attitudes and beliefs surrounding mental health within their peer groups.

Participants were recruited primarily through university email campaigns, local social media platforms (including Facebook, Reddit, and Craigslist), and the snowball method, whereby participants recommended additional subjects. This purposive sampling strategy was designed to approximate the demographic composition of young adults in the region. Fresno County's population is nearly evenly split by gender; accordingly, this study included sixteen women and fourteen men. In terms of ethnicity, 53.6 percent of Fresno County residents identify as Hispanic, and 60 percent of participants in this study were Hispanic. Similarly, 26.96 percent of locals are White, and 23.3 percent of the sample was White. Asians constitute 10.87 percent of Fresno County residents, and 10 percent of participants in this study identified as Asian. Finally, while 8.57 percent of the Fresno County population identifies as belonging to other racial or ethnic categories, 6.7 percent of participants in this study identified as being of Indian origin.

While this sample was designed to reflect the racial and gender demographics of young adults in Fresno County, "young adults" are anything but a uniform group. This age range includes people with vastly different lived experiences, including family situations, housing stability, income levels, and educational backgrounds. In part to protect a sense of trust and safety in my young adult subjects, I didn't collect detailed data on these kinds of first-space factors, so I cannot claim full generalizability across all young adult populations. Still, this diverse group offers grounded insight into how young adults from California's Central Valley, an often underrepresented and richly complex region, are thinking and feeling about media and mental health care access.

While the sample size (n = 30) limits the ability to make sweeping generalizations, the demographic composition reflects Fresno County and parallels broader state trends. These findings should be read as part of a larger conversation about how different young adult communities navigate care, and which messages are actually reaching them. The insights revealed through these interviews have value beyond the geographic range of the interviewee's home region. They can inform and influence communities and practitioners, even if they are not generalizable enough to be the sole driver of policy or practices. Future research could and should dig deeper into those socio-cultural layers and duplicate methods over larger subject sets to achieve greater generalizability.

The study received approval from Fresno State's Institutional Review Board (IRB), and all participants provided informed consent prior to participation. Interviews, conducted between June and December 2024, followed a semi-structured format. Each participant responded to the same set of questions in a consistent order, though I had the flexibility to ask follow-up questions for clarification or deeper insight. All interviews were conducted via Zoom, recorded, and transcribed using the Alice app. To protect confidentiality, all data were anonymized during transcription and analysis.

Participants answered eighty-seven questions, resulting in over 50,000 words of transcribed data. A critical content analysis was employed to identify recurring themes and validate findings across the dataset. Thematic analysis was conducted iteratively to ensure reliability and coherence. This analysis was partially guided by the TPB, which posits that human decision-making is guided by an interplay of social norms, efficacies (perceived behavioral control), and attitudes toward the behavior (Ajzen 1985).

While the study yields valuable insights, it has notable limitations. The sample size, while sufficient for qualitative analysis, may not fully capture the breadth of perspectives in the region. Furthermore, the snowball sampling method, although effective for reaching underrepresented populations, may have introduced selection bias. Lastly, conducting interviews online, while logistically convenient, may have influenced participant responses compared to in-person settings.

The full questionnaire is included in the appendix. For this study, "peers" were defined as individuals aged 18–25 years in the greater Fresno metro area. Media literacy skills were defined as the abilities to access, analyze, evaluate, create, and act using all forms of communication.

The Media Literacy Skills to Access, Evaluate, and Act on Mental Health Care Options

The vast majority of young adults feel like they have the skills they need to access mental health care, with 86.7 percent responding that they do. Additionally, the vast majority of young adults report having the skills to act on available mental health services, with 90 percent answering affirmatively to that question. Those who said no or maybe expressed concerns that they are too "shy" or "scared" to seek help.

Fewer young adults feel like they have the ability to evaluate the quality of those resources, with 40 percent of young adults saying they either don't have the skills or are not sure if they do. Some acknowledged not knowing what services they need because they don't know their own diagnosis and where to go from there. "I'm not so sure," said one young adult. "Especially when you're not sure of, like, what mental health services I necessarily need. That's, like, the big thing." Not having received care before is a limiting factor in being able to evaluate the quality of that care. "I have not used mental health resources, so I wouldn't be able to tell the difference," a young adult said. One young adult who answered no said, "I have been in therapy before, and I have learned that every therapist is not the right therapist for you. And that's okay. You know? It's okay not to like them or not. Maybe not to like them, but not to be, like, your vibe, I guess."

I asked young adults what media literacy skills they believe are essential for accessing available mental health care options. Using a critical content analysis approach, I compiled their responses into an outline that could serve as a foundation for developing a media literacy course curriculum or enhancing an existing one. The goal is to empower students to effectively navigate and utilize the care resources available to them. To ensure alignment with established factors that drive action, I organized the findings using the TPB framework.

Attitudes: Self-Awareness

According to the young adults I interviewed, individuals need to be able to recognize their own mental health challenges before seeking help. That self-awareness is the bridge between their internal worlds of emotions and thoughts, and the external world of media and information that is constantly impacting that internal world. "If you feel something, you're aware of it, then you might more be inclined to act on it rather than just be going through a certain negative emotion and just not really having any kind of awareness of that," as one subject said.

From a mental health care perspective, self-knowledge is critical for understanding what help is needed. "Tailoring the counseling to your specific needs is very crucial to the overall success of what (results) you want to get," said one young adult. "I think you need to be self-aware of what exactly you want. And reaching out to those specifically."

Attitudes: Less-Trusting Attitude Toward Sources

Young adults are often too quick to trust information presented to them online, according to those I interviewed. Young adults need to be taught "not just look at the first thing you see and believe that," as one subject put it, but "to be able to go through different options, whether it's like knowing what kind of website's reliable compared to what's not."

While they need to learn to differentiate professional resources (e.g., licensed therapists) from unverified advice, a critical foundational perspective is to be at least somewhat cynical about information that comes through social media, news, and entertainment content. "Advertising probably is just targeted towards you because of your clicks and everything," said one young adult, who urged their peers to seek help from valid resources like doctors. "Definitely being able to discern what could actually be beneficial for them and what is just someone, you know, saying something," as another subject put it.

Young adults talked about listening to content creators who talk about mental health but letting one's reaction to that content just be a first step, and not a perceived self-diagnosis. "Maybe if I feel a little bit stronger about the (content I'm seeing), I should probably talk to a health care professional or I should investigate a little bit more," said one young adult.

Young adults also mentioned the importance of consuming diverse media and verifying information through multiple sources, which highlights a belief that these actions lead to better understanding, critical thinking, and informed decision-making. "If you find something that interests you or something that sounds like something you would want to participate in or kind of do, you should probably look into it with more than just one thing," one young adult said. "Like, you shouldn't always just trust the first thing that you see." This relates to the sentiment young adults shared that researching something as important as mental health is not an immediate-gratification process. "I think they just need to put more time into what they're researching," said one subject.

Knowledge about common disorders and available support was also mentioned by multiple young adults. Knowledge about common disorders and available support shapes an individual's perception of mental health care as beneficial or necessary. "Just knowing which keywords to look for is the first step in media literacy," said one participant. Young adults were worried that others might hear an advertisement for a for-profit mental health care option without knowing there may be better treatment options available. "BetterHelp has been proven to be kind of shady to patients, and they don't have, like, the most qualified therapists working for them," said one young adult. "So being able to analyze a mental health care option or organization and see if they're genuine, I think is important."

Perceived Behavioral Control (Self-Efficacy)

Tech savviness and access were frequently mentioned, with a special emphasis placed on using a telephone as a critical efficacy that facilitates accessing mental health care, but which many young adults lack. "I find that making phone calls is easier to get in touch with, like, health care providers," one young adult said. Skills in using the telephone, email, and social media for research and outreach should all be emphasized, according to our young adults.

Research and evaluation skills were the most common skills mentioned in this data set. "I think research is a big part of media literacy and just kind of being able to know where to look to research is also pretty important," said one young adult. "Like, trusting valid websites and things like that for your sources." Or, as another young adult put it, "Check the sources." Numerous young adults stressed the skill of being able to distinguish between advertisements and genuine information as a critical skill on one's path to quality mental health care. Related to this skill is understanding algorithms and targeted content: "Just understanding what's more of an advertisement rather than something that can benefit you," as one subject put it. "Advertising probably is just targeted towards you because of your clicks and everything."

Social media posts by health care professionals can lead to informed decisions about mental health, reducing self-diagnosis and encouraging professional help. Evaluating this content is a skill. "There are a lot of scams out there," said a young adult, who also mentioned the fear of predators using sham resources to lure in victims. As another subject put it, "I think they should be able to do research into the organization or the research to see if this is actually like a company that's really going to help them or if it's a money grab or just something that isn't really there to help them."

This relates to actionable knowledge, or knowing how to act on resources through media channels. "I would probably teach them like how to find the like where to go like, because I don't know," said one young adult who portrayed the research skills needed to find care out of their reach. Other subjects encouraged media literacy educators to take a hand-holding approach. "I think walking students or kids through like how to practically do it instead of just preaching about like big concepts of like you need to critically think, but what does that actually look like?" one participant said. "I feel like walking them through like on your phone. 'Everyone pull out your phone We're gonna do like a demonstration type thing.'"

Critical thinking to evaluate personal needs was also mentioned by numerous young adults. Understanding when mental health content signals a need to get help relates to an individual's confidence and ability to perform a behavior, including having the necessary skills, knowledge, and tools. "Like the first thing that came to me when you said that was basically kind of like, critical thinking skills," one young adult said. "Kind of understanding how to, like, evaluate what it is that they need and then understanding how to apply that."

Nervous system regulation—or patience—was also presented as a foundational skill needed to access mental health care. "I think the skills (to access mental health care) should come from a little bit of emotional awareness and regulation awareness for sure," said one subject. Skills like self-regulation, taking the time to process information, and maintaining patience during research or decision-making are all needed to walk the long and winding road of media interactions on the way to sustained care. "We need a quick response with us," said one young adult of their generation's disposition. "They go through text or they don't have the patience to even just call someone."

Subjective Norms

Young adults need to understand how social stigma and cultural perceptions impact their attitude toward mental health and mental health care. Stigma, young adults understand, can be a barrier to individuals seeking help: "A lot of mental health disorders are stigmatized, and as a result, these people aren't able to get help because they'll see people post about these mental health disorders and they feel discouraged to even seek help in the first place," said one young adult. Negative perceptions discourage help-seeking behavior. "It can be kind of hard to get people to access mental health help when their families are so against it," said one young adult. "Like, there's really big stigmas against mental health in Mexican homes. It doesn't get taken seriously at all."

The role of supportive therapists and peers is a critical element in young adults' mental health journeys. Participants stressed that empathetic and engaging counselors are fundamental to the success of treatment, as they help individuals feel understood and valued. One participant shared, "I think having a counselor therapist that is understanding and very empathetic is so crucial." Another added, "If you're not engaged with what your counselor is saying, it's hard. It's kind of like a teacher—if the teacher's just rambling and out of control, it's hard to maintain focus."

In addition to professional support, peer connections play a significant role in encouraging individuals to seek help. One participant noted, "The ability to reach out to other people and ask" is a valuable skill, emphasizing the importance of having accessible and supportive social networks. Similarly, fostering relatable experiences in safe spaces can make seeking help feel more approachable: "Maybe the students will be like, 'Oh, I've been through that, so maybe I could get the help of [a counselor].'"

How—and from Whom—Young Adults Want to Receive Information About Available Mental Health Care

I asked young adults whom they want to receive information about available mental health care services from, among the following options: social media, news outlets, fliers/posters, other media outlets such as television, film, or podcasts, your professors, family members, or peers. The overwhelming response was that they want to hear from friends and peers (70 percent), followed by professors (50 percent), family 46.67 percent, and social media (26.67 percent). Nothing else received more than two mentions. The young adults were very clear that they want to receive this information from people they know.

"That's who I trust the most, and they know me the most, so I feel like they would give me respected opinions," one young adult said. "I trust everyone in my circle, and if they think that's what's best for me, I appreciate that information from them because I have a lot of trust and respect with them," another said. "If they're suggesting it, that means it's probably what's in my best interest." Hearing from people like them who have already been down the road of care helps. "Definitely peers, because I feel like they could, you know, give me their own experiences with those specific resources," another young adult said.

I also asked young adults whether they would prefer to receive information about available mental health care services through video, podcast/audio, in written form, through virtual reality, or in person, the most popular answer, by far, was in person, with 50 percent of young adults saying this is their preferred method of receiving information about mental health care. As one subject put it, "I would prefer in person because I find that whenever I talk to someone face to face, it's a lot easier for me to sort of relate to what they're talking about and, like, take it in better," they said. "When someone is getting information, say, at home or on their phone, there's a lot of distractions going on already." Others emphasized the trust one can gain from an interpersonal interaction. "Just because it's like the human connection," one said. "There's nothing like a human connection." While several subjects mentioned podcasts being a preferred method, they also recognized that with podcasts or videos, it can be easy to just swipe to the next piece of content and skip the part about available mental health care.

I asked the young adults a similar question, but without option prompts (for reference, this question came much earlier in the survey than the responses to the above question). When asked how they want to receive information about available mental health care services, there were only three organic responses mentioned by the young adults: 46.67 percent said in person, 30 percent said over email, and 20 percent said via social media. Once again, young adults referenced the safety they feel through human interaction. "I think one on one conversations and hearing it from other people and testimonials is very helpful," said one young adult who had already accessed services. "I feel that's what really got me into the program." Again, young people referenced their attention spans as a limiting factor when it comes to receiving information through any media at all. "Like, I hate doing the work sometimes," one said, "If I get presented something and I'm like, 'Okay, I'll take the time to at least pay attention if it's there in front of me.'" Another benefit of receiving this information in-person, young adults said, is that it offers the opportunity to ask questions.

What mediums have already been effective in reaching young adults with information about available mental health care options? When asked if they could recall times in the past year when they were exposed to information about mental health care services and through which medium, 73.33 percent recalled encountering such information through entertainment media, 63.33 percent through fliers or posters, and another 63.33 percent through social media (see Table 5.1) Numerous young adults mentioned the ubiquitous BetterHelp advertisements that have popped up in their social media feeds.

Beyond the survey data, interview responses also underscored the impact of face-to-face encounters. In an open-ended part of the interview process, 40 percent of young adults recalled being exposed to mental health care information in person. There was something about learning about these services face-to-face that seemed to stick. "I get them like all the time, like random emails (about care)," said one young adult. "They don't really hit as well for me as seeing someone in person and being able to talk and ask them questions. It really helped me out and it actually inspired me to go there and see what they had to offer."

The Mediums that Reach Them: The Media Young Adults Like, Trust, and Would Utilize to Access Mental Health Care

Next, I present a quantitative snapshot of the data to provide a broad overview of how young adults in the Fresno metro currently perceive various media channels. It is important to note that the interview questions were not presented in a multiple-choice format. Instead, responses were open-ended and subsequently categorized by the researcher into predefined coding categories. Due to the relatively small sample size, the data was not further disaggregated by sex or race. This analysis is intended to offer a general cultural perspective rather than detailed, actionable insights about specific demographic subgroups within the young adult population.

These results highlight the appeal of TikTok, which 93.33 percent of young adults call easy to use, and that 76.67 percent of young adults say they plan to use in the near future. The majority of respondents find TikTok to be useful for accessing mental health care information (53.33 percent), and two-thirds say they will use it to access mental health care information. When asked if there is a social media platform they believe is best positioned to reach young adults with information about mental health care services, TikTok was the clear favorite, mentioned by nineteen of the thirty respondents (63.33 percent). Despite

Table 5.1 Comprehensive Analysis of Mental Health Access Barriers, Facilitators, and Media Literacy Skills Across Young Adults

Question	% Positive/Yes	% Negative/No	% Maybe/Sometimes/Unsure
Do you consider social media platforms to be reliable suppliers of information related to available mental health care services?	30	16.67	53.33
Do you recall receiving information about available mental health care services through any social media platforms?	63.33	36.67	0
Do you believe social media platforms should be sharing information about available mental health care services?	100	0	0
What is your attitude toward TikTok?	43.33	30	26.67
Do you believe your peers use or watch TikTok?	100	0	0
Do you know how to use TikTok?	83.33	16.67	0
Do you believe it to be easy to use?	93.33	6.67	0
Do you intend to use this in the near future, in general?	76.67	20	3.33
Do you intend to use it to access available mental health care services?	66.67	26.67	6.67
Is this medium useful for accessing mental health care information?	53.33	30	16.67
What is your attitude toward Instagram?	73.33	23.33	3.33
Do you believe your peers use Instagram?	100	0	0
Do you know how to use Instagram?	96.67	3.33	0
Do you believe it to be easy to use?	96.67	3.33	0
Do you intend to use this in the near future, in general?	93.33	3.33	3.33
Do you intend to use it to access available mental health care services?	53.33	33.33	13.33

Question	% Positive/Yes	% Negative/No	% Maybe/Sometimes/Unsure
Is this medium useful for accessing mental health care information?	66.67	20	13.33
What is your attitude toward Twitter/X?	20	70	10
Do you believe your peers use Twitter/X?	60	10	30
Do you know how to use Twitter/X?	80	17	3
Do you believe it to be easy to use?	77	13	10

Do you intend to use this in the near future, in general?	40	57	3
Do you intend to use it to access available mental health care services?	6.67	86.67	6.67
Is this medium useful for accessing mental health care information?	30	40	30
What is your attitude toward Facebook?	33.33	50	16.67
Do you believe your peers use Facebook?	36.67	50	13.33
Do you know how to use Facebook?	73.33	23.33	3.33
Do you believe it to be easy to use?	73.33	16.67	10
Do you intend to use this in the near future, in general?	50	50	0

Question	**% Positive/Yes**	**% Negative/No**	**% Maybe/Sometimes/Unsure**
Do you intend to use it to access available mental health care services?	16.67	73.33	10
Is this medium useful for accessing mental health care information?	46.67	20	33.33
What is your attitude toward Snapchat?	10	56.67	33.33
Do you believe your peers use Snapchat?	73.33	20	6.67
Do you know how to use Snapchat?	93.33	6.67	0
Do you believe it to be easy to use?	100	0	0
Do you intend to use this in the near future, in general?	30	66.67	3.33
Do you intend to use it to access available mental health care services?	0	96.67	3.33
Is this medium useful for accessing mental health care information?	10	73.33	16.67
What is your attitude toward local TV news?	50	36.67	13.33
What is your attitude toward local digital/print news media, like the *Fresno Bee*?	63.33	20	16.67
Do you believe your peers watch local TV news?	13.33	73.33	13.33
Do you believe your peers read local digital/print news media?	20	66.67	13.33

(*Continued*)

Table 5.1 (*Continued*)

Question	% Positive/Yes	% Negative/No	% Maybe/Sometimes/Unsure
Do you intend to watch local TV news in the near future?	56.67	36.67	6.67
Do you intend to watch local TV news to access information about available mental health care services?	43.33	56.67	0
Do you intend to read local digital/print news in the near future?	53.33	36.67	10
Do you intend to read local digital/print news to access information about available mental health care services?	43.33	46.67	10
Do you consider local news outlets to be reliable suppliers of information related to available mental health care services?	70	10	20
Do you recall receiving information about available mental health care services through any local news outlets?	6.67	90	3.33
Do you believe local news outlets should be sharing information about available mental health care services?	100	0	0
What is your attitude toward films, TV, podcasts, and YouTube?	100	0	0
Do you believe you have the ability to access and use these forms of media?	100	0	0
Do you intend to consume films, TV, podcasts, or YouTube in the near future?	100	0	0
Do you intend to consume films, TV, podcasts, or YouTube in the near future for the purpose of accessing available mental health care services?	53.33	33.33	13.33
Do you consider entertainment content—such as film, television series, podcasts, and YouTube—to be reliable suppliers of information related to available mental health care services?	56.67	10	33.33
Do you recall receiving information about available mental health care services through any forms of entertainment content?	73.33	26.67	0

Question	% Positive/Yes	% Negative/No	% Maybe/Sometimes/Unsure
Do you believe entertainment media companies should be sharing information about available mental health care services?	93.33	3.33	3.33
What is your attitude toward fliers and posters?	60	20	20
Do you read them?	40	23.33	36.67
Do you believe your peers read fliers and posters?	43.33	33.33	23.33
Do you intend to read fliers and posters?	63.33	16.67	20
Do you intend to seek out information about mental health care services from fliers and posters?	60	23.33	26.67
Do you consider fliers and posters to be reliable suppliers of information related to available mental health care services?	73.33	3.33	23.33
Do you recall receiving information about available mental health care services through fliers or posters?	63.33	33.33	3.33
What is your attitude toward email newsletters?	50	40	10
Do you read them?	46.67	3.33	20
Do you believe your peers read email newsletters?	30	30.67	33.33
Do you intend to read email newsletters?	53.33	26.67	20
Do you intend to seek out information about mental health care services from these sources?	40	36.67	23.33

Question	% Positive/Yes	% Negative/No	% Maybe/Sometimes/Unsure
Do you consider email newsletters to be reliable suppliers of information related to available mental health care services?	50	6.67	43.33
Do you recall receiving information about available mental health care services through email newsletters?	23.33	60	16.67

enthusiastically negative responses toward TikTok by some young adults, who called it "addicting," "brain rot," and "a waste," it still appears to reign supreme in the local young adult social media landscape.

The only social media that appeared as or more appealing as a medium for mental health care information was Instagram, which 93.3 percent of young adults said they would use in the near future. Young adults feel that more humanity comes through the video format. "You actually get to see the person," a subject said. "You get to hear their voice. You actually get to, like, *hear* someone." More than half of young adults said they would use this social media to access mental health care services, and two-thirds said it is useful for accessing mental health care information. Seventeen young adults said Instagram is the social media best positioned to reach young adults (56.57 percent). Young adults like that Instagram allows for multiple slides per post, which makes it easy to include actionable information. According to one young adult, "From what I've seen on Instagram, it kind of has that hook in where it's like, 'Hey, we're getting legitimate resources out to you, but we're making it fun and like cool to be a part of.'"

Young adults cited a sense of justice that social media apps like Instagram should share information about available mental health care services. "Instagram, not only does it create a lot of beauty standards, it's the cause of people's low self-esteem," a young adult said. "I think by having that balance of also promoting mental health and mental health awareness, it's just like, it's a nice balance."

Facebook and Snapchat were the lesser two popular of the four social media apps we asked about. Only a third of respondents have a positive outlook on Facebook, while only 10 percent have a positive perspective on Snapchat. Only 16.67 percent of young adults plan to use Facebook to access available mental health care, with 0% planning to use Snapchat. Only 10 percent of young adults said that Snapchat is useful for accessing mental health care information. Facebook was cited by numerous young adults as being a place for older adults, while conversely, Snapchat was framed as being for a younger generation.

* * *

The study shows that young adults have a mixed relationship with local news. Over 63 percent of respondents have a positive attitude toward local print news, such as the *Fresno Bee*. Seventy percent of young adults find print/digital news outlets to be reliable suppliers of information related to mental health car services. "Because I think as a local source, they probably have the information said one young adult, who echoed a common refrain that the localness of news makes it more trustworthy. "They may have a connection or network to vouch for the available options in the area."

Yet, only 6.67 percent of young adults could recall receiving information about mental health care services through these mediums. When asked if there is a local news outlet they believe is best positioned to reach young adults with information about mental health care services, nine young adults mentioned ABC30, five said the *Fresno Bee*, and four said *Fresnoland*.

When asked what advice they have for local news outlets that might have a goal of reaching young adults with mental health care information, respondents stressed that they prefer to see peers or individuals close to their age sharing stories or promoting resources, and they want to see personalized success stories. They want news organizations to provide direct links and clear contact information for where they can access care, and any news content related to mental health needs to be shared via social media, where young adults are more likely to receive it. "Stay consistent" with the content "and don't be cringey (be real)" were themes mentioned by multiple young adults.

* * *

In terms of reaching young adults in the media where they are (and say they will be), nothing can beat entertainment media, which includes YouTube, podcasts, films, and television. 100% of young adults surveyed have a positive view of entertainment media, and 100% of them plan to consume it in the near future. Most respondents said they plan to seek out information about mental health care options through entertainment media, and the majority considered entertainment outlets to be reliable sources of this information.

"Nothing better than hearing it from an influencer or content creator that is going through the same struggles as the everyday people and can share their experiences and let people realize, hey, it's okay to go through this," said one young adult. Subjects noted that their favorite entertainment content creators can inspire them to seek mental health help. "They do encourage you to, if you're struggling with the same issues, to look for help and give you the resources or a list to kind of start looking into. As opposed to just, 'this is what I'm struggling with. I'm keeping it to myself.'" Knowing someone who has gone through something similar—even through a parasocial relationship with someone the [illegible]t will never meet—can facilitate care. "Hearing that somebody that has gone through it makes you feel a little bit more personal to it, more likely to reach out to those resources," a young adult said.

A notable 73.33 percent of young adults can recall receiving information about mental health care through entertainment media—mostly BetterHelp through podcasts or YouTube—which speaks to the ubiquity of mental health-related advertisements on these sites, along with possibly a higher retention rate of these interactions when they happen while consuming entertainment media. The more entertainment media companies talk about mental health and mental health care, the more mainstream it becomes for all, subjects said. More sharing of resources "would lower the stigma and open and increase the likelihood for people to seek treatment or therapy or disinformation about mental health," a young adult said. "And right now, because it isn't as covered, I feel like it creates a cycle of mental health illness still being a stigma which reduces people's likelihood to seek treatment."

When asked what advice they would give entertainment media companies that hope to reach more young adults with mental health care information, young adults want them to focus on stories, keep it short, link to resources, and most of all, keep it real. "Just to come off as genuine about it and not like you're meeting some sort of quota of, like, being woke about mental health," said one young adult. As much as possible, young adults want the stories and the care to be specific to them and where they're from. "I would just say try to make the advertisements like specific, you know, and like catered towards your actual group that you're going for," a young adult said. "Like if you're going for Fresno State students who live in Fresno County, you know, when you're showing off the information, show Victor Bulldog, you know, show, show some like other stuff that maybe people can relate to."

When asked if there is a film/TV/podcast or YouTube channel they believe is best positioned to reach young adults with information about mental health care services, young adults had no shared specific answers but frequently cited YouTube and podcasts, where mental health care communicators can place their ads within content that is relevant.

* * *

Despite being known as a more traditional medium, young adults are receptive to fliers. Sixty percent of young adults have a positive attitude toward fliers, 63.33 percent said they intend to read fliers, 73.33 percent consider fliers to be reliable forms of this kind of information, and 63.33 percent recall receiving information about available mental health care through fliers or posters. The comment made repeatedly by young adults was that design is everything when it comes to whether they notice a flier. "If they look cool, I like to look at them," one subject said. "It has to be eye catching," said another. "If it catches my eye," "If it catches my attention," and "if the design is cool" were other representative responses. "It depends on how good the posters are," a subject said. "If they're just text and not a lot of colors, not a lot of shapes on it, we're kind of like monkeys with it. It's like, all right, I'm not reading that." Young adults like that on fliers it can be quick and easy to tell if a source is credible, based on an organizational logo, and they like that QR codes can take them directly to where they need to go to get help.

Finally, email newsletters are read by a minority of young adults (46.67 percent), but half of young adults consider these to be a reliable source of mental health care-related information, and numerous others consider them trustworthy when they trust the source. "Annoying but useful," was a representative response. Young adults like that email newsletters can feel more personalized. "I think that most times people with email blasts do know your audiences," a subject said. "So, you know, like if it's a school one, if they're going to give you information for students by students on campus. Or I went to some women's retreat and they say, hey, sign up for this because we're going to let you know about the next one. They know who I am, they know my age, they know, you know, that I'm there, why I'm there, what I care about."

How to Reach Us: Direct Feedback from Young Adults to Promoters of Mental Health Care Options

When asked what grade level information about available mental health care should be written in to reach virtually every member of their peer group, a third of young adults said ninth grade, while a third said even younger, answering middle school or even elementary school, and six said eighteen years old.

When asked what languages this information should be available in, virtually all young adults said both English and Spanish. Multiple other languages were mentioned, including Hmong, Vietnamese, Punjabi, Japanese, Arabic, and Hindi, with Hmong and Punjabi mentioned the most. Overall, young adults believe this information should be available in all the languages used in their region. "Any language that's probably spoken predominantly around the area where I'm in," as one young adult put it.

When asked what mental health care communicators need to understand about the culture of their peers to reach them with information about available mental health care, the young adults shared a similar set of themes to what we've already encountered. I distilled these responses into the five most commonly referenced themes.

Their Attention Spans Are Debilitatingly Short

Interviewee after interviewee referenced the limitation of their short attention spans. With young adults, it's all about the first five seconds they're exposed to something. "You got to catch their attention in the first five seconds," said one young adult. "If you don't catch their attention in the first five, ten seconds, I'm just gonna scroll up." Young adults speculated about universal ADHD among their generation, "so in that little attention span of information, (you have to give us) something that's more digestible than something long."

Mental health communicators should know they're competing for attention with the other media young adults are exposed to. "A lot of our lives involves social media and being on our phones," a young adult said. "We need a reason to stop and look at it." One young adult went into more detail:

> So I think they need to understand that people want their information fast. If they were to look at an email, they want to know, like, the main benefits right away. They don't want to, like, you know, have to, like, dig deep to figure out every little thing. I'd say if they were to send an email or do any sort of social media advertisement, they should have everything clearly labeled right at the front. . . . Like, here's what you have available to you and this is why you should do it. Like, boom, boom, boom. Like, if there's some way to summarize it all, like, within a sentence or two for each, like, service, that would be a good way of going about it.

They Have Trust Issues; They're Scared

Young adults don't necessarily feel safe in the realm of mental health care and mental health-related conversations. "They should understand that most of them are probably not cool with other people knowing, like, their peers knowing that they need mental health," said one young adult, echoing the commonly referenced theme of not feeling safe to share or reach out for help. "We have major trust issues," said one young adult. "It's mostly trust issues. Sometimes we don't trust any adult at all. (If we don't trust mental health care communicators) it's because we don't trust our parents."

There was a fear that counselors may expose what they share to family or peers. "I feel like, you know, everyone's anxious about putting themselves out there," one subject said. "Or embarrassed, like, 'Oh, someone's gonna record me, and I'm gonna look stupid.'"

A lack of MHL and a lack of understanding of the health care system raise anxieties. "It's very hard to start that first step," one young adult said. "So whatever help they can do (to help at the first step), do it."

The mental health issues themselves become functional barriers to care. "I think people that are kind of holding that stuff inside are generally more shy, more anxious, I guess," said one young adult. "I think the biggest hurdle for somebody that is in need of help is just making the first step. Telling somebody that they need help, being vulnerable."

There are those who are too afraid to express that they are mentally or emotionally unwell. "A lot of people hide their feelings, so they never seek help," a young adult said.

Stigma Has Stuck Around

Functionally speaking, stigma leads to denial. "Many people don't think they need help," said a young adult. "But they do. They don't think they need it because they don't want to feel crazy. Let them know that just because you have a mental issue doesn't mean you're crazy."

Stigma was common within the families of the young adults interviewed. "My dad, he is very much like he would see someone on the news who maybe committed suicide or something like that. He'd be like, 'Oh, it's because they're just crazy,'" one young adult said. "It's just gonna be harder to reach those communities because they're not gonna feel like what they're going through is valid because their families don't think it's valid already."

Many participants referenced cultural attitudes, especially within Hispanic and older-generation communities, as significant barriers to discussing and addressing mental health. "Well, I'm Mexican, and I grew up in, like, a super Mexican town," said a young adult from the greater Fresno region. "Like, it's probably 98 plus percent Mexican, and in a lot of Mexican households, I know a lot of my friends, like, their parents don't believe in mental health. They don't think it's real. So it can be kind of hard to get people to access mental health help when their families are so against it."

Stigma was referenced beyond just the Hispanic respondents. It remains a universal concern. "They should understand that as much as there is less stigma within our age group, there still is the presence of stigma," said one young adult. "So we really need to focus on making it cool to talk about. And again, that goes back to it being aesthetically artistically digestible and having more people within our age group be the messengers talking about it, not teachers that are, you know, 15, 20 years older."

Content Needs to Be Relatable, and Relate to Different Cultures in Different Ways

"Make it immediately relatable," said one young adult.

Young adults highlighted the diversity of cultures within their generation, emphasizing that even different age ranges within the group have distinct mindsets. As one participant noted, "They need to find a way that reaches people in those certain ages because 18 year olds can have a different mindset compared to those that are 25 years old. So having that relatability when reaching out to those certain age groups is crucial."

Participants consistently emphasized the importance of having resonant messengers—people from the same age group and with relatable cultural touchstones—deliver mental health messages to increase trust and resonance. "I think it really depends on the community that you're trying to target when it comes to young adults," said one subject. "It might be bringing up something that is trendy right now or, like, following the trends. Like, TikTok videos or even commercials, they start off with something or a sound that might be trending. Or if there is a picture of something that they've seen before, it catches their attention."

A critical audience to diversify for is those impacted by stigma. "Being aware of understanding that there's going to be different positions on mental health, and not assuming that everyone in my generation is going to be like, 'Oh, yes, we support mental health,'" said one young adult. And not everything needs to be humorous. "People of my generation group do take things seriously," said one young adult. "So not everything has to be like funny or anything like that or lik almost made like a joke."

It could help, at least one young adult speculated, to have people of their generation making the mental health-related content intended to reach them. As one young adult put it:

> I think those, like, mental health care companies, I think, should hire people from my generation because there's no one better to understand what my group is going through than someone who's actually in it, instead of just seeing, like, middle aged people trying to figure out, like, trying to think that they know what this group is going through when they don't. So having someone my age group can relate to, I think that would be a great step in the right direction.

They're Hurting but They're Not Necessarily Being Open About It

"A lot of people hide their feelings, so they never seek help," said a young adult, echoing one of the most common themes of the data set. "A lot of people are really struggling and they could probably use some help," said another.

Dotted across interviews were references to the quiet suffering among themselves and their peers. "We're chronically online, whether it's beneficial or damaging, and we're not always open to speaking up about what we're going through," stated one interviewee.

A spirit of independence can work against young adults who need mental health care.

"I feel like I've noticed in my generation, a lot of people are, like, kind of quiet about what they may be going through and have the mentality of, like, 'I can fix this myself.'"

"I feel like, you know, everyone's anxious about putting themselves out there," said another young adult.

Conclusion

Recommendations and Reflections

The primary aim of this project was to enhance our understanding of how media serves as a conduit to mental health care for American young adults, in order to increase mental health care access through better media literacy practices and awareness. This demographic is amid a mental health crisis, yet many are not accessing the care they need. In California, only 37 percent of adults with mental illness received mental health services in the previous year, compared to a national average of nearly 43 percent (Wiener 2019). Young adults are deeply embedded in media ecosystems, where access to care is often just a few clicks away. However, significant gaps remain in reaching this population effectively and in equipping them with the skills to identify and act upon opportunities for care.

A media literacy framework offers a critical avenue for addressing these issues. We can bridge these gaps by analyzing the expectations placed on mental health communicators and empowering educators to teach media literacy skills. This approach not only facilitates more effective communication but also empowers young adults to navigate and leverage available resources for their mental well-being.

The recommendations outlined in this conclusion, derived from the original research collected in Chapters 3 and 4 and supported by the literature, are directed toward American policymakers, educators, and mental health professionals. These findings themselves are not revolutionary, but a focus on the intersection of media literacy and mental health care is a novel way of increasing mental health care access in our communities. By fostering more efficient pathways for information and support, we can better connect young adults in need with the resources and care providers equipped to help them reclaim their mental health and well-being. By enhancing the clarity, relevance, and dissemination of mental health information, institutions can establish more equitable and effective pathways to support. In doing so, we can reduce systemic barriers and more effectively connect young adults with the services necessary to restore and maintain their mental health.

Mental Health Care Communicators

On a practical level, mental health care communicators should *keep it simple, keep it personal, and grab their audience within the first five seconds*, as young adults readily acknowledge that their attention spans can be limited. This echoes the work of Pretorius and their team, whose study of digital pathways to mental health care for young people recommended the key design considerations of accessibility, personalization, immediacy, and connectedness (Pretorius et al. 2020).

Mental health care communicators should know that the young adults they are trying to reach might have a low or nonexistent MHL and vocabulary, and *communicators should build education on foundational mental health concepts into their promotions*. This is vital, as higher MHL is a known facilitator of care (Aguirre Velasco et al. 2020), and in some cases has been shown to predict the use of therapy (Bonabi et al. 2016). Increasing MHL can help bolster several factors related to access, including reducing stigma toward professional help, building self-efficacy, and improving attitudes toward help-seeking (Suwanwong et al. 2024). The help-seeking process for mental health issues starts with awareness, knowledge, recognition, and an evaluation of symptoms—all of which are bolstered by higher MHL (Gagnon et al. 2017).

Mental health care communicators should keep the core TPB principle of self-efficacy in mind and *offer clear step-by-step guidance on how to access care*, with first-timers particularly kept in front of mind. The hardest step is often the first step, as many of our interviews emphasized. It is wise for those of us with overlapping privileges of mental health literacy, health care systems literacy, and media literacy to reflect on how confusing numerous aspects of the initial steps to care can be for those without these privileges. As previous research has shown, young people with higher MHL are more likely to believe that suggested treatments will work and are more likely to seek professional help in the first place (Wright et al. 2012). It is not enough to tell young adults about available mental health care; we have to teach them about mental health care—and how to access it.

Promotion should happen in-person whenever possible, which was the clear preference of those interviewed for these studies. It is how young adults say they want to receive information about mental health care options. It is how they remember having received that information. It is what the mental health promoters interviewed here have witnessed as the most effective method. There is more mistrust of the mental health system among young adults than I expected to be revealed by this research. The bond created by in-person promotion, particularly when it is peer-to-peer, seems to be a magic code that unlocks the gate to the pathway to care. Peer-led mental health promotion interventions on college campuses have been shown to lead to significant increases in mental health awareness and knowledge of coping strategies, including formal care (Ahorsu et al. 2021). A systemic umbrella review of the effectiveness of peer support approaches for mental health that spanned 40,927 participants found that peer support can be effective at improving some clinical outcomes, self-efficacy, and recovery (Cooper et al. 2024). Personally, I believe we are designed to heal within community. Mental health promoters should be innovating ways to scale peer-to-peer outreach to emphasize the human connection that so many of our young adults are missing.

Outreach strategies must be thoughtfully diversified to effectively engage each target culture. There is a clear "need for improved policies and culturally relevant evidence-based interventions in improving mental health seeking attitudes and overall care, specifically for underserved populations" (Yirenya-Tawiah and Cubbin 2025, 1). For example, one of America's campuses' most pressing public mental health needs exists in the Native/Alaska Native community, whose screening levels for depression jumped from about a third in 2016 to over half in 2019–20, outpacing other ethnic and racial groups (Lipson et al. 2022). According to this research, being Native meant to be part of the group with the largest increases in suicidal ideation, depression, and anxiety. Being Native meant to be part of the group that experienced the largest decrease in flourishing. "There has not been nearly enough research on this population," Lipson told Boston University's *The Brink* (Colarossi 2022). "My hope is that these data document the urgency around understanding some of the unique factors shaping these students' mental health. American Indian/Alaska Native students need to be brought into the conversation for universities to invest in resources that align with their preferences."

Certain at-risk groups have been disproportionately affected by the mental health crisis. For example, Arab Americans have experienced a 22 percent increase in mental health prevalence alongside an 18 percent decrease in treatment utilization (Lipson et al. 2022). Expecting a single mental health marketing campaign to resonate equally with hedonistic atheists from Berkeley and practicing Muslims from Jordan is unrealistic. As other research has made clear, individuals struggled to engage with non-culturally sensitive health services (Stepanova et al. 2025). As Stepanova and their team recommended, "Culturally sensitive mental health services need to be integrated into existing systems through initiating collaborations with ethnic minority communities that tailor services to meet the needs of diverse populations, improving overall engagement and experiences" (1). Each cultural and ethnic group requires tailored approaches that consider their unique contexts and needs.

Distinct ethnic and cultural groups *should be invited to actively participate in the development of mental health communication strategies*. These communities must be directly involved in crafting messages that serve as the bridge between those in need and the care available to them. As Alang (2019) found, there is a "need for mental health systems to seek and take seriously the perspectives of people who experience unmet need" (362). Hines and their team recommended that to have culturally responsive mental health services, those offering care should, "collaborate with community and cultural brokers to change the narrative about seeking therapy or counseling" (Hines et al. 2023, 7). While mental health stigma exists in nearly every culture, its manifestations are unique to each. Consequently, stigma must be understood and addressed in culturally specific ways to create effective outreach and intervention strategies.

The ultimate goal is culture-specific messaging that is pushed through the media that culture most trusts and accesses, leading to care that is adapted to that culture. It is asking a lot, but it is what our students of color, queer students, and other minority groups need and deserve as, "the lack of inclusive and language-specific treatment options might constitute a structural obstacle for minority populations" (Molander et al. 2024).

A *data-driven approach to efficiency should extend to reflecting on how communication and media strategies are successfully—or unsuccessfully—reaching specific populations and need groups*. The American Council on Education recently published the report *What Works for Improving Mental Health in Higher Education* (Abelson et al. 2023). Authored by investigators from the Healthy Minds Study, this report synthesized findings from a variety of academic fields and journals to evaluate the effectiveness of campus mental health interventions. The report's foremost recommendation is to "use data to regularly assess population-level needs, priorities, and progress" (PDF p. 6). Abelson and their team further advocated for analyzing data on barriers to accessing mental health services and support. Or, as Okolo and their team put it, "By harnessing the power of data analytics, researchers and healthcare practitioners can design more effective, tailored communication strategies that ultimately improve health outcomes and reduce disparities across communities" (Okolo et al. 2024, 1435). These barriers may sometimes be rooted in gaps within the communication pathways between those providing services and the individuals who need them most.

We still have to devote energy to mental health stigma eradication and the normalization of conversations about mental health and mental health care, as stigma remains a formidable barrier for young populations (Villatoro et al. 2023). The young adults and mental health communicators I interviewed were clear about this. Mental health communicators need to be aware of stigma in their messaging, particularly with college students, 41 percent of whom believe that most people would think less of someone who has received mental health treatment (Eisenberg et al. 2023). The research about reaching young men still echoes in my ears: they are more receptive to mental health-related information when getting help is framed as them leaning into their masculine strengths (Sagar-Ouriaghli et al. 2019).

Mental health communicators should remain aware of the fact that trust can be low in the mental health system among young adults. Trust emerged as a recurring theme in both my interviews and the literature, consistently identified as a pivotal factor in determining whether young adults seek care or avoid it. In health communication, trust is as valuable as it is difficult to cultivate (Aguirre Velasco et al. 2020), and trust has been shown to increase help-seeking in young people (Meadley et al. 2024). Increasing mental health and mental health systems literacy is a way of increasing trust. For example, young people are most likely to have positive attitudes about mental health seeking when they expect confidentiality following disclosure (DeLuca 2018). Young adults may need to be explicitly told about state and national laws related to confidentiality and explicitly informed about the provider's confidentiality policies and practices.

Mental health care communicators should tap into the power of peers whenever possible to reach young adults, as expressed by young adults, mental health providers, and communicators interviewed, and supported by the literature. Effective interpersonal relationships are essential for fostering self-disclosure, as demonstrated by Calear and colleagues in their trial of an Australian peer connectedness school-based program aimed at promoting help-seeking behaviors in adolescents (Calear et al. 2022). Their research highlighted the unique potential of peer-to-peer networks, especially in disadvantaged areas where connections to trusted adults may be limited. Family dynamics and cultural norms often hinder open discussions about mental health among young adults, who may find peers to be a more empathetic audience (Liu and Zhang 2024).

Peer support interventions have shown consistently positive results across various modalities. Peer support can open up members to different types of experiences, build a support network, and improve symptoms (Thomson et al. 2024). A review of seventeen studies evaluating peer support as a tool for improving mental health outcomes in young adults found these interventions increase happiness, self-esteem, and coping skills, while reducing depression, loneliness, and anxiety (Richard et al. 2022). Notably, these effects were observed not only in university students but also in non-student young adults and ethnic or sexual minorities.

The amplification of positive social norms, increased self-efficacy, and improved attitudes among peers creates a ripple effect that the formal mental health care community alone cannot replicate. Peer support plays a vital role in expanding access to mental health care by providing empathetic, community-based support outside formal clinical systems (Sim and Choo 2025). Peer support has been shown to have largely positive effects on the mental health outcomes of young adults as they relate to depressive symptoms, anxious symptoms, psychological distress, and self-esteem (Richard et al. 2022). It is possible that peer interactions can be "gamified" to induce better results. Researchers exploring an online game designed to lower barriers to mental health care access suggested incorporating collaborative information-sharing features, such as social networking services, to facilitate the creation and maintenance of new support networks (Shandley et al. 2010).

Given the existing prevalence of online communities, *mental health interventions may find the greatest efficiency by meeting young adults where they already digitally gather*. "There is potential for mental health service providers to tap into the support already being provided by online communities," wrote Mitchell et al. (2017, 9) in their review of young adult help-seeking behaviors. They further noted, "As online and mobile services become more integrated with our everyday lives, so too will they become more integrated with the provision of mental health services" (9). Pretorius and their team echoed these findings in the systematic review of young people and their online help-seeking for mental health difficulties, saying, "Key benefits included anonymity and privacy, immediacy, ease of access, inclusivity, the ability to connect with others and share experiences, and a greater sense of control over the help-seeking journey. Online help-seeking has the potential to meet the needs of those with a preference for self-reliance or act as a gateway to further help-seeking" (Pretorius et al. 2019, 1).

Media Literacy Educators (and Educators at Large)

American media literacy educators should continue to emphasize foundational digital literacy skills, including research, analysis, and media creation. The goal here is not to redirect the full scope of media literacy education toward mental health access. Rather, it is to highlight how media literacy can be strategically leveraged to support young adults in developing the digital competencies necessary to navigate and access available mental health resources. Exploring this intersection presents a valuable opportunity to enhance both media literacy outcomes and public health impact.

Educational institutions that serve young adults need to take greater responsibility for addressing the disconnect between students and available mental health care. At all levels, schools must ensure that students leave equipped with the skills to access these critical services. MHL interventions in schools have shown they can improve attitudes around help-seeking (Nazari et al. 2024). The CDC has advised that school systems and educators take the lead, noting that schools can increase students' MHL by delivering classroom-based mental health education curricula and implementing peer-led modeling programs (Centers for Disease Control and Prevention 2023). Educators need to step in where parents are unprepared. According to a 2023 California Health and Human Services report, parents expressed that a lack of information, resources, and support limited their understanding of behavioral health challenges and their ability to provide support. This played a role in 65 percent of young people with depression going without mental health treatment due to a lack of access to services (California Health and Human Services Agency 2023). The obligation to address mental health care access among young adults extends to public school systems with mandated media literacy education and to colleges that have increasingly incorporated media literacy courses, including the university where I teach, Fresno State University.

The good news is that quality media literacy education can play a significant role in bridging the mental health care access gap, offering not just understanding but healing. As Suwanwong and their team found in their systematic review of potentially modifiable predictors of MHL in the educational context, "educational institutions can cultivate communities adept in mental health, fostering an environment marked by empathy, understanding, and proactive engagement in addressing mental health issues" (2024, 378). Program quality is paramount. Hayes et al. (2024), in their systematic review of fourteen school-based interventions designed to improve help-seeking, evaluated their quality using the Effective Public Health Practice Project tool. Unfortunately, most interventions were rated as low quality, highlighting the need for robust and well-designed initiatives to ensure meaningful outcomes.

A growing body of research emphasizes that educational institutions should play a leading role in preparing young adults to effectively access mental health care. "Higher education is fundamentally designed to understand and address complex challenges, and its leaders now have the opportunity and responsibility to improve how we support the mental health and well-being of students," argue the authors of *What Works for Improving Mental Health in Higher Education* (Abelson et al. 2023, 16). Yet, according to the Healthy Minds Study, which surveyed over 500,000 college students, only 6 percent reported receiving counseling or emotional support from a faculty member or professor (Lipson et al. 2022). Considering the amount of face time professors have with students—particularly those in their majors—this disconnect demands further investigation.

The gap between student needs and expectations is stark. Nearly half of students believe professors should play a role in supporting mental health, according to the 2023 Student Voice survey, which involved a nationally representative sample of 3,000 undergraduates across 158 institutions (Flaherty 2023). Despite these expectations, the availability of supportive adults is declining. A 2022–3 YouthTruth survey of over 500,000 high school students found that only 41 percent felt they had an adult at school they could talk to about mental health issues, a drop from 46 percent in the decade preceding the pandemic (YouthTruth 2024). The authors described this "support gap" as striking.

Professors, however, are well-positioned to serve as conduits to care. A Dutch study highlighted the role of school personnel and peers in positively influencing help-seeking behaviors, emphasizing the importance of recognition, encouragement, and easy access to providers (Eigenhuis et al. 2021). Outside the home, schools are often where mental health concerns are first identified. "Young people spend most of their day at school interacting with adults and peers, all of whom can be empowered to connect those in need to early intervention and treatment supports," writes the New Hampshire Department of Education (n.d., 1). Universities are also uniquely positioned to act as hubs for addressing mental health concerns originating in their environments, particularly when offering comprehensive financial and academic accommodations (Liu and Zhang 2024).

Untreated mental health issues can significantly hinder students academically, affecting attention, problem-solving, homework completion, and test performance, among other areas (New Hampshire Department of Education n.d.). A study of almost 2,000 Japanese college students found that impaired mental health status in the first semester significantly predicts an increased risk of poor academic performance throughout their undergraduate education (Chu et al. 2022). Conversely, another study found that digital literacy can mediate the relationship between emotional intelligence and academic stress (Ibrahim et al. 2024). Addressing these issues benefits the entire school community. "Young people who receive appropriate mental health supports have improved academic achievement . . . and are more likely to attend and successfully complete college," notes the Substance Abuse and Mental Health Services Administration (2019, 2).

The social, emotional, and academic development of young people is strengthened in schools that offer comprehensive mental health resources and are staffed with trained professionals equipped to support the diverse needs of the student population (Wriston et al. 2023). "In the big picture, we need to bring mental health into the classroom so that it doesn't require a student needing to make time or getting motivated to seek help," explains Sarah K. Lipson of the Healthy Minds Network (Colarossi 2022). Lipson emphasizes the need to make mental health support a default part of students' lives. Research underscores the importance of non-familial youth-adult relationships in mental health promotion programs. Jagosh et al. (2024) describe how such relationships foster collective agency and relationally embedded opportunities for youth to explore their ideas and lead systems transformation. By creating "Third Space and Third Place counterspaces," adult facilitators provide environments for young people to build adaptive responses, broaden their communities, and pursue personal change.

Mental health education should be carefully integrated with media literacy education to address critical gaps in young people's ability to access and optimize mental health care. Although media literacy education and health education may seem like unlikely partners, they are, in fact, complementary. For example, "helping young people to assign credibility to online resources also has the potential to play an important role in developing their mental health literacy," Pretorius and their team wrote (Pretorius et al. 2020, 5). MHL is not enough without media literacy, as was exhibited through a study of nursing students—who we can assume have high health literacy—and how social media use related to depression. The authors found that, "problematic social media use and low mental health literacy are significant risk factors for depression, and their interaction significantly increases the risk" (Jiayuan et al. 2025). Together, media literacy and MHL equip young adults with the skills to navigate their paths to care and make informed decisions.

Mental health education provides media-literate young adults with the tools to identify what to seek when they need care and to interpret the "road signs" on their way to finding it. Both media literacy and health literacy are essential for accessing and optimizing care. For instance, media savvy alone is insufficient if a young adult cannot distinguish between the short-term relief of anxiety-related social media content and the long-term benefits of professional treatment from a licensed clinician. Conversely, possessing high health literacy without media literacy is equally limiting in a world increasingly driven by digital platforms—akin to knowing how to drive without access to a car. Wharf Higgins and Begoray (2012) developed the construct of Critical Media Health Literacy in 2012, defining CMHL as "a right of citizenship and empowers individuals and groups, in a risky consumer society, to critically interpret and use media as a means to engage in decision-making processes and dialogues; exert control over their health and everyday events; and make healthy changes for themselves and their communities" (142). As defined by these researchers, CMHL recognizes that in order to increase the public's skills at accessing mental health care, it is imperative to address their ability to access and interpret health information from various sources, including websites, mass media, health education pamphlets, family, and friends.

Levin-Zamir and Bertschi (2018) more recently described critical media health literacy as the ability to identify health-related messages in the media, recognize their potential influence on health behaviors, critically analyze their content, and apply the information to one's own health decisions—including accessing available mental health care (1). In their study of CMHL in online college students, Squires and their team concluded that "educating students to be more critical of the information consumed online, especially when it is health-related, can impact overall wellness and health-compromising or health-promoting behaviours" (Squires et al. 2023, 68).

The stakes of media literacy education (or the lack thereof) can be striking, particularly when it comes to mitigating the mental health risks associated with media consumption and empowering young people to analyze, access, and act on health care options. Misinformation can be deadly. "Social media poses a threat to public health by facilitating the spread of misinformation," Walter and colleagues observed in their meta-analysis of health misinformation online (Walter et al. 2021, 1776). Young people commonly use social media to learn about mental health, where they are often met with misinformation, which can lead to dangerous self-diagnosis and attempts to meet their needs in unhealthy ways (Rizwan and Weigle 2025). Poor MHL is associated with higher rates of depression, anxiety, stress, internalized stigma, and caregiver burden, and in today's highly mediated world, it is challenging if not impossible to have MHL without media literacy (Tambling et al. 2023).

The profound impact of media on mental health underscores the necessity of dedicating substantial portions of media literacy courses to mental health topics. Both qualitative data from interviews and existing literature support this approach. For instance, research demonstrates that larger positive emotion vocabularies are associated with higher well-being and better physical health (Vine et al. 2020). Similarly, a significant positive correlation has been found between emotional vocabulary size, emotional granularity, and mental health outcomes (Ikeda 2023).These findings highlight the vital role of emotional and media literacy in fostering resilience and well-being in young people. As numerous young adults and mental health providers pointed out, media literacy education also needs to encompass self-regulation and self-awareness education if we want it to improve access to mental health care. Patience is not just a virtue; it is a vital skill one needs to thoroughly research any important issue in one's life, be it political or mental health care access. Self-awareness and self-regulation are foundational media literacy skills, and others are already seeing them as such. In Kosic's (2018, 83). research on the opportunities of combining media literacy and social-emotional literacy, they found that "media literacy training and explicit socio-emotional teaching empowers young people to engage actively in their own learning to develop their life skills and competencies," including the efficacy to access available mental health care.

Educators must empower young people to become their own mental health advocates. Media literacy education can empower young adults to leverage media to benefit their own health (Weinstein and James 2022). As one mental health care promoter from the Fresno metro area remarked, “Friends and family like to tell you what to do. Only you know what you should do.” This highlights the importance of equipping individuals with the skills and confidence to navigate their mental health journeys independently.

The continuum from a young adult realizing they need care, to utilizing media to access care, to actually getting to and sticking with care, is rife with potential speed bumps and pitfalls (Ådnanes and Steihaug 2013). What happens when a campaign successfully leads someone to a therapy modality or practitioner that isn’t right for them? Finding the appropriate therapy, practitioner, medium, and setting is rarely a straightforward process, and is often quite fragmented for young adults (Modi et al. 2022). “Getting help” often involves multiple decisions, including a series of deflating *No*’s before a final, empowering *Yes*, with many falling through the gaps in the process (Appleton et al. 2022). This underscores the need to teach young adults to be champions of their own healing. “Emotions are complex. You can’t just blanket treat things anymore,” a mental health promoter explained to me. They encouraged young adults to, “Go out there and listen [to what’s available and what’s going on with yourself]. It’s not just feeling sad. It’s so much deeper than that.” It goes deeper, and the road to the right care might be long enough that resilience and self-motivated leadership are necessities to ensure access.

The final verb in the NAMLE definition of media literacy is the ability to *act* using all forms of communication (National Association for Media Literacy Education, n.d.a). Media literacy educators must teach students not only how to navigate modern media landscapes but also how to use media assertively, with confidence and efficacy, to promote their own mental wellness, health, and financial well-being. This critical step—acting—goes beyond what is typically required in most high school or college courses. It demands leaving the confines of the classroom and taking actionable steps, such as booking a first counseling appointment.

“Everyone has a really complicated relationship with media,” observed Michelle Lipkin, NAMLE’s executive director, in a personal interview. “And that’s why what I love about media literacy education is it affords us the opportunity to have those deeper conversations.” Media literacy education can, and should, create a space for students to engage with media on a personal level, fostering the skills and confidence necessary for self-advocacy in mental health and beyond.

State Legislators and School Boards

All media literacy educators should receive formal training in media literacy education. This training must be mandated, funded, and accessible, as currently we are seeing states pass media literacy laws that don't include training mandates or funding (Langreo 2022). Media literacy pedagogy and skill development should be a required component of K–12 teacher preparation programs, ensuring that educators possess both the knowledge and skills to effectively teach this vital subject. Some studies suggest that teachers are entering the media literacy classroom feeling under-prepared (Gretter and Yadav 2018). Continuing education will be necessary to help educators keep pace with the rapid evolution of media technologies, shaped by Silicon Valley and Hollywood innovations, as teachers already are not confident in their ability to teach competencies related to media creation and participatory media skills (McNelly and Harvey 2021).

This media literacy training should extend beyond educators to encompass other professionals who regularly interact with adolescents and young adults. Educators cannot address the critical gaps in mental health care access on their own. The 2023 report by the National Academies of Sciences, Engineering, and Medicine on minimizing the harms and maximizing the benefits of social media for adolescent health recommends that "accrediting bodies for the education of doctors, nurses, and social workers should incorporate training on the effects of social media on child and adolescent health into curricula" (National Academies of Sciences, Engineering, and Medicine 2023). This recommendation is crucial, but I would expand the scope to include mental health care workers and mental health care promoters. Moreover, the training should go beyond social media effects to provide a comprehensive understanding of media effects, information theories, media industries, and media creation. Media—and particularly social media—is deeply woven into the fabric of adolescent and young adult experiences. Health care professionals must move beyond a bystander understanding of these technologies to develop an active, nuanced perspective that equips them to address the complexities of media's influence on mental health and well-being.

I encourage elected officials to consider how media and especially social media can be mandated to help increase access to available mental health care through their channels. I encourage elected officials to consider mandating digital versions of warning labels that educate young people on the potential risks of consuming that media on their mental health and well-being. These media and social media companies that are playing distinct roles in harming the mental health of our young adults should be warning them and attempting to help them.

* * *

We have the capacity—and the responsibility—to do better for our young adults who are suffering from mental health issues. This body of research lays clear that we can improve mental health care access through more aware media literacy education and practices, along with mental health care promotion that better considers how young adults interact with the media that can be the bridge to care.

References

ABC30. 2022a. "Fresno County Sees a Drop in Deaths by Suicide." *ABC30 News*, February 22, 2022. https://abc30.com/fresno-county-suicide-stats/11526698/.

ABC30. 2022b. "The Diabetes Epidemic in the Central Valley." *ABC30 News*, August 2, 2022. https://abc30.com/diabetes-central-valley-fresno-county-merced/12001488/.

Abelson, Sara, Sarah Ketchen Lipson, and Daniel Eisenberg. 2023. *What Works in College Mental Health?*. American Council on Education. https://www.acenet.edu/Documents/What-Works-Mental-Health.pdf.

Abrams, Zara. 2022. "Student Mental Health Is in Crisis. Campuses Are Rethinking Their Approach." *Monitor on Psychology*, October 12, 2022. https://www.apa.org/monitor/2022/10/mental-health-campus-care.

Adams, Claire, Eyal Gringart, and Natalie Strobel. 2022. "Explaining Adults' Mental Health Help-Seeking through the Lens of the Theory of Planned Behavior: A Scoping Review." *Systematic Reviews* 11 (1): 160. https://doi.org/10.1186/s13643-022-02034-y.

Adams, Claire, Eyal Gringart, Natalie Strobel, and Paul Masterman. 2021. "Help-Seeking for Mental Health Problems Among Older Adults with Chronic Disease: An Application of the Theory of Planned Behaviour." *Australian Journal of Psychology* 73 (4): 426–37. https://doi.org/10.1080/00049530.2021.1952850.

Ådnanes, Marian, and Sissel Steihaug. "Obstacles to Continuity of Care in Young Mental Health Service Users' Pathways – An Explorative Study." *International Journal of Integrated Care* 13 (July–September 2013): e031. https://doi.org/10.5334/ijic.1135

Aguirre Velasco, Antonia, Ignacio Silva Santa Cruz, Jo Billings, Magdalena Jimenez, and Sarah Rowe. 2020. "What Are the Barriers, Facilitators, and Interventions Targeting Help-Seeking Behaviours for Common Mental Health Problems in Adolescents? A Systematic Review." *BMC Psychiatry* 20: 293. https://doi.org/10.1186/s12888-020-02659-0.

Ahorsu, Daniel Kwasi, Aghdas Haghayegh, Reza Rostami, Chung-Ying Lin, Mark D. Griffiths, Amir H. Pakpour, and Ramin Mojtabai. 2021. "Effect of a Peer-Led Intervention Combining Mental Health Promotion with Coping-Strategy-Based Workshops." *International Journal of Mental Health Systems* 15 (1): 3. https://doi.org/10.1186/s13033-020-00432-0.

Ajzen, Icek. 1985. "From Intentions to Actions: A Theory of Planned Behavior." In *Action Control: From Cognition to Behavior*, edited by Julius Kuhl and Jürgen Beckmann, 11–39. Springer-Verlag.

Alang, Seena M. 2019. "Mental Health Care Among Blacks in America: Confronting Racism and Constructing Solutions." *Health Services Research* 54 (2): 346–55. https://doi.org/10.1111/1475-6773.13115.

Albano, Teresa. 2021. "Illinois Becomes the First State to Require Media Literacy Classes for High School Students." *The Progressive*, August 31, 2021. https://progressive.org/latest/illinois-first-state-media-literacy-albano-210831/.

Aldalaykeh, Mohammed, Mohammed M. Al-Hammouri, and Jehad Rababah. 2019. "Predictors of Mental Health Services Help-Seeking Behavior Among University Students." *Cogent Psychology* 6 (1): 1660520. https://doi.org/10.1080/23311908.2019.1660520.

Ali, Kathina, Daniel B. Fassnacht, Louise Farrer, Elizabeth Rieger, Johannes Feldhege, Markus Moessner, Kathleen M. Griffiths, and Stephanie Bauer. 2020. "What Prevents Young Adults from Seeking Help? Barriers Toward Help-Seeking for Eating Disorder Symptomatology." *International Journal of Eating Disorders* 53 (5): 894–906. https://doi.org/10.1002/eat.23266.

Allcott, Hunt, Matthew Gentzkow, and Lena Song. 2022. "Digital Addiction." *American Economic Review* 112 (7): 2424–63. https://doi.org/10.1257/aer.20210867.

Alonso, Jordi, Michael C. Angermeyer, Silvia Bernert, Ron de Graaf, Maria Isabel Bruffaerts, Jean-Pierre Brugha, Gemma Bryson, et al. 2004. "Prevalence of Mental Disorders in Europe: Results from the European Study of the Epidemiology of Mental Disorders (ESEMeD) Project." *Acta Psychiatrica Scandinavica Supplementum* 109 (420): 21–7. https://doi.org/10.1111/j.1600-0047.2004.00327.x.

Amado-Rodríguez, Isaac Daniel, Rocio Casañas, Laia Mas-Expósito, Pere Castellví, Juan Francisco Roldan-Merino, Irma Casas, Lluís Lalucat-Jo, and Mª Isabel Fernández-San Martín. 2022. "Effectiveness of Mental Health Literacy Programs in Primary and Secondary Schools: A Systematic Review with Meta-Analysis." *International Journal of Environmental Research and Public Health* 19 (7): 4199. https://doi.org/10.3390/children9040480.

American College Health Association. 2023. *National College Health Assessment III: Spring 2023 Reference Group Executive Summary.* Accessed December 9, 2024. https://www.acha.org/documents/ncha/NCHA-III_Spring_2023_Reference_Group_Executive_Summary.pdf.

American College Health Association. 2024. *Student Health Data from the Spring 2024 NCHA Now Available.* https://www.acha.org/news/student-health-data-from-the-spring-2024-ncha-now-available/.

American Foundation for Suicide Prevention. 2024. "Suicide Statistics." *AFSP.* Accessed December 3, 2024. https://afsp.org/suicide-statistics.

Anteola, Bryant-Jon. 2021. "Fresno Is California's Most Dangerous City to Drive Due to Drunk Drivers, Study Says." *The Fresno Bee*, November 13, 2021. https://www.fresnobee.com/news/local/article255695276.html.

Antoniou, Georgia, Emilie Lambourg, J. Douglas Steele, and Lesley A. Colvin. 2023. "The Effect of Adverse Childhood Experiences on Chronic Pain and Major Depression in Adulthood: A Systematic Review and Meta-Analysis." *British Journal of Anesthesia* 130 (6): 729–46. https://doi.org/10.1016/j.bja.2023.03.008.

Appleton, Rebecca, Joelle Loew, and Faraz Mughal. 2022. "Young People Who Have Fallen through the Mental Health Transition Gap: A Qualitative Study on Primary Care Support." *British Journal of General Practice* 72 (719): e413–20. https://doi.org/10.3399/BJGP.2021.0678.

Aschbrenner, Kelly A., Stephen J. Bartels, Kristin L. Naslund, Sarah E. Tomlinson, Alexandra Kinney, Susan I. Pratt, and Mary F. Brunette. 2019. "Adolescents' Use of Digital Technologies and Preferences for Mobile Health Coaching in Public Mental Health Settings." *Frontiers in Public Health* 7: 178. https://doi.org/10.3389/fpubh.2019.00178.

Ashley, Seth, Adam Maksl, and Stephanie Craft. 2017. "News Media Literacy and Political Engagement: What's the Connection?" *Journal of Media Literacy Education* 9 (1). https://digitalcommons.uri.edu/jmle/vol9/iss1/6/.

Astridge, Belinda, Wendy Wen Li, Brett McDermott, and Carlo Longhitano. 2023. "A Systematic Review and Meta-Analysis on Adverse Childhood Experiences: Prevalence in Youth Offenders and Their Effects on Youth Recidivism." *Child Abuse & Neglect* 139: 105737. https://doi.org/10.1016/j.chiabu.2023.105737.

Aufderheide, Patricia. 1993. *Forum Report: Media Literacy. A Report of The National Leadership Conference on Media Literacy, The Aspen Institute Wye Center, Queenstown, Maryland, December 7–9, 1992.* American University.

Austin, Erica W., Bruce W. Austin, Jessica Fitts Willoughby, Ofer Amram, and Shawn Domgaard. 2021. "How Media Literacy and Science Media Literacy Predicted the Adoption of Protective Behaviors Amidst the COVID-19 Pandemic." *Journal of Health Communication* 26 (4): 239–53. https://doi.org/10.1080/10810730.2021.1899345.

Austin, Erica W., Bruce W. Austin, Porismita Borah, Shawn Domgaard, and Sterling M. McPherson. 2022. "How Media Literacy, Trust of Experts, and Flu Vaccine Behaviors Are Associated with COVID-19 Vaccine Intentions." *American Journal of Health Promotion* 37 (4): 464–70. https://doi.org/10.1177/08901171221132750.

Bandura, Albert. 1986. *Social Foundations of Thought and Action: A Social Cognitive Theory*. Prentice-Hall.

Bantjes, Jason. 2022. "Digital Solutions to Promote Adolescent Mental Health: Opportunities and Challenges for Research and Practice." *PLOS Medicine* 19 (5): e1004008. https://doi.org/10.1371/journal.pmed.1004008.

Bas, Gokhan. 2020. "Relation between Student Mental Health and Academic Achievement Revisited: A Meta-Analysis." In *Behavioral Neuroscience*, edited by Fatima Shad Kaneez. IntechOpen. https://doi.org/10.5772/intechopen.94368.

Beck, Jonathan S., Rebecca A. Lundwall, and Mikle South. 2020. "Looking Good but Feeling Bad: 'Camouflaging' Behaviors and Mental Health in Women with Autistic Traits." *Autism* 24 (4): 809–21. https://doi.org/10.1177/1362361320912147.

Beltramini, Richard F., and Patrick D. Bridge. 2001. "Relationship between Tobacco Advertising and Youth Smoking: Assessing the Effectiveness of a School-Based Antismoking Intervention Program." *Journal of Consumer Affairs* 35 (2): 263–77. https://doi.org/10.1111/j.1745-6606.2001.tb00116.x.

Benedetto, Lucia, and Maria Ingrassia. 2021. "Digital Parenting: Raising and Protecting Children in Media World." In *Parenting: Studies by an Ecocultural and Transactional Perspective*, 127–48. IntechOpen.

Berkman, Nancy D., Terry C. Davis, and Lauren McCormack. 2010. "Health Literacy: What Is It?" *Journal of Health Communication* 15 (sup2): 9–19. https://doi.org/10.1080/10810730.2010.499985.

Bhui, Kamaldeep, and Dinesh Bhugra. 2002. "Mental Illness in Black and Asian Ethnic Minorities: Pathways to Care and Outcomes." *Advances in Psychiatric Treatment* 8 (1): 26–33. https://doi.org/10.1192/apt.8.1.26.

Bhushan, Devika, Kristen Kotz, Jacey McCall, Sherry Wirtz, Ruth Gilgoff, Shanta R. Dube, Christine Powers, Julie Olson-Morgan, Maria Galeste, Kristine Patterson, Louise Harris, Ashley Mills, Christina Bethell, Nadine Burke Harris, and Office of the California Surgeon General. 2020. *Roadmap for Resilience: The California Surgeon General's Report on Adverse Childhood Experiences, Toxic Stress, and Health.* Office of the California Surgeon General. https://doi.org/10.48019/PEAM8812.

"Bill Text – AB-873 Pupil Instruction: Media Literacy." 2024. *California Legislative Information*. https://leginfo.legislature.ca.gov/faces/billNavClient.xhtml?bill_id=202320240AB873.

Birkley, E. L., C. I. Eckhardt, and R. E. Dykstra. 2016. "Posttraumatic Stress Disorder Symptoms, Intimate Partner Violence, and Relationship Functioning: A Meta-Analytic Review." *Journal of Traumatic Stress* 29 (5): 397–405. https://doi.org/10.1002/jts.22129.

Bohon, Lisa M., Kelly A. Cotter, Richard L. Kravitz, Philip C. Cello Jr., and Erik Fernandez y Garcia. 2016. "The Theory of Planned Behavior as It Predicts Potential Intention to Seek Mental Health Services for Depression among College Students." *Journal of American College Health* 64 (8): 593–603. https://doi.org/10.1080/07448481.2016.1207646.

Bonabi, Herdis, Mario Müller, Vladeta Ajdacic-Gross, Jochen Eisele, Stephanie Rodgers, Erich Seifritz, Wulf Rössler, and Nicolas Rüsch. 2016. "Mental Health Literacy, Attitudes to Help Seeking, and Perceived Need as Predictors of Mental Health Service Use." *The Journal of Nervous and Mental Disease* 204 (4): 321–4. https://doi.org/10.1097/NMD.0000000000000488.

Borah, Porismita, Erica Austin, and Yan Su. 2022. "Injecting Disinfectants to Kill the Virus: Media Literacy, Information Gathering Sources, and the Moderating Role of

Political Ideology on Misperceptions about COVID-19." *Mass Communication and Society* 25 (4): 523–45. https://doi.org/10.1080/15205436.2022.2045324.

Botts, Jackie, Byrhonda Lyons, and Erica Yee. 2024. "A Breakdown of California's Mental Health System, Explained." *CalMatters*. Accessed December 3, 2024. https://calmatters.org/explainers/breakdown-californias-mental-health-system-explained/.

Bryant, Ashleigh, Amy Cook, Helen Egan, Jeffrey Wood, and Michail Mantzios. 2021. "Help-Seeking Behaviours for Mental Health in Higher Education." *Journal of Further and Higher Education* 46 (4): 522–34. https://doi.org/10.1080/0309877X.2021.1985983.

Burke, Lauren, Mary John, and Paul Hanna. 2022. "A Qualitative Exploration of How Young Men in the UK Perceive and Experience Informal Help-Seeking for Mental Health Difficulties." *Children and Youth Services Review* 136: 106440. https://doi.org/10.1016/j.childyouth.2022.106440.

Burnette, C. Blair, Melissa A. Kwitowski, and Suzanne E. Mazzeo. 2017. "'I Don't Need People to Tell Me I'm Pretty on Social Media': A Qualitative Study of Social Media and Body Image in Early Adolescent Girls." *Body Image* 23: 114–25. https://doi.org/10.1016/j.bodyim.2017.09.001.

Byrne, D. G., S. C. Davenport, and J. Mazanov. 2007. "Profiles of Adolescent Stress: The Development of the Adolescent Stress Questionnaire (ASQ)." *Journal of Adolescence* 30 (3): 393–416. https://doi.org/10.1016/j.adolescence.2006.04.004.

Calear, Alison L., Michelle Banfield, Philip J. Batterham, Alyssa R. Morse, Owen Forbes, Bradley Carron-Arthur, and Martin Fisk. 2017. "Silence Is Deadly: A Cluster-Randomised Controlled Trial of a Mental Health Help-Seeking Intervention for Young Men." *BMC Public Health* 17: 834. https://doi.org/10.1186/s12889-017-4845-z.

Calear, Alison L., Philip J. Batterham, Michelle Torok, and Sonia McCallum. 2021. "Help-Seeking Attitudes and Intentions for Generalised Anxiety Disorder in Adolescents: The Role of Anxiety Literacy and Stigma." *European Child & Adolescent Psychiatry* 30 (2): 239–49. https://doi.org/10.1007/s00787-020-01512-9.

Calear, Alison L., Sonia M. McCallum, Helen Christensen, Andrew J. Mackinnon, Alexandra Nicolopoulos, Jacqueline L. Brewer, Aliza Werner-Seidler, Alyssa R. Morse, Dominique Kazan, Louise M. Farrer, Laura Kampel, and Philip J. Batterham. 2022. "The Sources of Strength Australia Project: A Cluster Randomised Controlled Trial of a Peer-Connectedness School-Based Program to Promote Help-Seeking in Adolescents." *Journal of Affective Disorders* 299: 435–43. https://doi.org/10.1016/j.jad.2021.12.012.

California Department of Education. n.d. "Media Literacy Resources." Accessed December 19, 2024. https://www.cde.ca.gov/Ci/cr/ml/index.asp.

California Health and Human Services Agency. 2023. "Youth at the Center: Outcomes and Insights from the Youth-Centered Design Process." *CHHS*. https://www.chhs.ca.gov/wp-content/uploads/2023/01/CYBHI-Youth-at-the-Center-Report.FINAL_.pdf.

California Health Care Foundation. 2024. "New 2024 California Health Care Foundation Survey." Accessed December 7, 2024. https://www.chcf.org/press-release/new-2024-chcf-ca-health-policy-survey/.

California State Legislature. 2023. *AB-873 Pupil Instruction: Media Literacy: Curriculum Frameworks (2023–2024)*. October 16, 2023. https://leginfo.legislature.ca.gov/faces/billTextClient.xhtml?bill_id=202320240AB873.

"California to Teach Media Literacy in Every Grade." 2023. *Assemblymember Marc Berman*. October 14, 2023. https://a23.asmdc.org/press-releases/20231014-california-teach-media-literacy-every-grade.

Campion, Jonathan, Kamaldeep Bhui, and Dinesh Bhugra. 2012. "European Psychiatric Association (EPA) Guidance on Prevention of Mental Disorders." *European Psychiatry* 27 (2): 68–80. https://doi.org/10.1016/j.eurpsy.2011.10.004.

Canizales, Stephanie L. 2019. "Potential Stressors of Undocumented Latinx College Students: An Integrative Review." *Hispanic Journal of Behavioral Sciences* 41 (2): 151–73. https://doi.org/10.1177/0739986319837180.

Center for Collegiate Mental Health. 2023. *2023 Annual Report*. Pennsylvania State University. Accessed December 9, 2024. https://ccmh.psu.edu/assets/docs/2023_Annual%20Report.pdf.

Centers for Disease Control and Prevention. n.d. "Youth Risk Behavior Surveillance System (YRBSS): Data Summary & Trends Report." Accessed December 8, 2024. https://www.cdc.gov/yrbs/dstr/index.html.

Centers for Disease Control and Prevention. 2023. *Promoting Mental Health and Well-Being in Schools: An Action Guide for School and District Leaders*. US Department of Health and Human Services. https://www.cdc.gov/mental-health-action-guide/media/pdfs/DASH_MH_Action_Guide_508.pdf.

Center for Media Literacy. n.d. "Resources for Educators." Accessed December 19, 2024. https://www.medialit.org/.

Chen, Guo-Ming. 2007. "Media (Literacy) Education in the United States." *China Media Research* 3 (3): 87–94. http://www.wwdw.chinamediaresearch.net/index.php/back-issues?id=35.

Chen, Shu-Ping, Michelle Koller, Terry Krupa, and Heather Stuart. 2016. "Contact in the Classroom: Developing a Program Model for Youth Mental Health Contact-Based Anti-Stigma Education." *Community Mental Health Journal* 52 (3): 281–93. https://doi.org/10.1007/s10597-015-9944-7.

Cho, Hyunyi, Julie Cannon, and Wenbo Li. 2022. "Social Media Literacy: A Conceptual Framework." *New Media & Society* 26 (2): 340–57. https://doi.org/10.1177/14614448211068530.

Chu, Tianshu, Xin Liu, Shigemi Takayanagi, Tomoko Matsushita, and Hiro Kishimoto. 2022. "Association between Mental Health and Academic Performance among University Undergraduates: The Interacting Role of Lifestyle Behaviors." *International Journal of Methods in Psychiatric Research* 32 (1): e1938. https://doi.org/10.1002/mpr.1938.

Coffman, Janet. 2022. *An Overview of California's Behavioral Health Workforce.* Healthforce Center, Philip R. Lee Institute for Health Policy Studies, University of California, San Francisco. July 12. https://hcai.ca.gov/wp-content/uploads/2022/07/Agenda-Item-9-HCAI-HWET-Council-07-12-2022_Final-ADA-Accessible.pdf.

Colarossi, Jessica. 2022. "Mental Health of College Students Is Getting Worse." *BU Today*, April 21. https://www.bu.edu/articles/2022/mental-health-of-college-students-is-getting-worse/.

Coles, Meredith E., and Shannon L. Coleman. 2010. "Barriers to Treatment Seeking for Anxiety Disorders: Initial Data on the Role of Mental Health Literacy." *Depression and Anxiety* 27 (1): 63–71. https://doi.org/10.1002/da.20620.

Common Sense Media. 2022. *The Common Sense Census: Media Use by Tweens and Teens.* https://www.commonsensemedia.org/sites/default/files/research/report/8-18-census-integrated-report-final-web_0.pdf.

Community Health System. 2022. *2022 Community Health Needs Assessment.* September 19, 2022. https://www.communitymedical.org/getmedia/79018eb4-f102-4932-bd43-78378afee64f/CommunityHealthSystem_2022CHNA_9-19-22.pdf.

Community Medical Centers. n.d. "Early Intervention, Support Important for Treating Mental Disorders." Accessed December 13, 2024. https://www.communitymedical.org/about-us/newsroom/early-intervention-important-for-mental-disorders.

Compton, Josh, Ben Jackson, and James A. Dimmock. 2016. "Persuading Others to Avoid Persuasion: Inoculation Theory and Resistant Health Attitudes." *Health Communication* 31 (2): 140–50. https://doi.org/10.1080/10410236.2015.1035176.

Condo, Pat. 2023. "Just 3 States Require Teaching Media Literacy. Growth of AI Makes It Essential." *The 74 Million*, October 10, 2023. https://www.the74million.org/article/just-3-states-require-teaching-media-literacy-growth-of-ai-makes-it-essential/.

Cooper, Ruth E., Katherine R. K. Saunders, Anna Greenburgh et al. 2024. "The Effectiveness, Implementation, and Experiences of Peer Support Approaches for Mental Health: A Systematic Umbrella Review." *BMC Medicine* 22: 72. https://doi.org/10.1186/s12916-024-03260-y.

County of Fresno Behavioral Health. 2024. "Multi-County Suicide Prevention Summit." *Facebook*, December 13, 2024. https://www.facebook.com/reel/435640799385774.

County of Fresno Department of Behavioral Health. 2021. "MENtal Health Campaign Launches to Address Mental Health Stigma Among Men." Accessed December 1, 2024. https://www.facebook.com/Fresnocountybehavioralhealth/posts/have-you-seen-our-newest-effort-to-addressing-mental-health-stigma-and-promote-w/988572119437486/.

Czeisler, Mark É., Rashon I. Lane, Emily Petrosky, Joshua F. Wiley, Annie Christensen, Rashid Njai, Michael D. Weaver, Rebecca Robbins, Emma R. Facer-Childs, Laura K. Barger, Charles A. Czeisler, Mark E. Howard, and Shantha M. W. Rajaratnam. 2020. "Mental Health, Substance Use, and Suicidal Ideation During the COVID-19 Pandemic—United States, June 24–30, 2020." *Morbidity and Mortality Weekly Report* 69: 1049–57. https://doi.org/10.15585/mmwr.mm6932a1.

Dalton, Madeline A., James D. Sargent, Michael L. Beach, Linda Titus-Ernstoff, Jennifer J. Gibson, M. Bridget Ahrens, Jennifer J. Tickle, and Todd F. Heatherton. 2003. "Effect of Viewing Smoking in Movies on Adolescent Smoking Initiation: A Cohort Study." *The Lancet* 362 (9380): 281–5. https://doi.org/10.1016/S0140-6736(03)13970-0.

de Sá, Vitor Rabelo, Paula Victoria Sozza Silva Gulá, Tamiris Prizon, Raquel Messi Falcoski, Rafael Naime Ruggiero, and Fernando E. Padovan-Neto. 2023. "Anxiety and Functional Impairment Affects Undergraduate Psychology Students' Learning in Remote Emergency Teaching During the COVID-19 Pandemic." *Scientific Reports* 13: 27845. https://doi.org/10.1038/s41598-023-27845-4.

Deloitte Access Economics. 2020. *The Social and Economic Cost of Eating Disorders in the United States of America: A Report for the Strategic Training Initiative for the Prevention of Eating Disorders and the Academy for Eating Disorders.* June. https://www.hsph.harvard.edu/striped/report-economic-costs-of-eating-disorders/.

DeLuca, Joseph S. 2018. "Conceptualizing Adolescent Mental Illness Stigma: Youth Stigma Development and Stigma Reduction Programs." *Adolescent Research Review* 3 (3): 293–308. https://doi.org/10.1007/s40894-018-0106-3.

Division of Student Affairs and Enrollment Management. 2023. *Annual Report 2023.* Fresno State. https://studentaffairs.fresnostate.edu/documents/annual-report-23.pdf.

Doll, Carolin M., Chantal Michel, Marlene Rosen, Naweed Osman, Benno G. Schimmelmann, and Frauke Schultze-Lutter. 2021. "Predictors of Help-Seeking Behaviour in People with Mental Health Problems: A 3-Year Prospective Community Study." *BMC Psychiatry* 21: 432. https://doi.org/10.1186/s12888-021-03435-4.

Duthie, Grant, Nicola Reavley, Judith Wright, and Amy Morgan. 2024. "The Impact of Media-Based Mental Health Campaigns on Male Help-Seeking: A Systematic Review." *Health Promotion International* 39 (4): daae104. https://doi.org/10.1093/heapro/daae104.

Edegoh, Leonard O., Blessing O. Asemah, and Monday N. Ezebuenyi. 2022. "Social Media Literacy and Youth Digital Citizenship in Nigeria: Implications for Policy and Practice." *Social Science Research* 103: 102582. https://doi.org/10.1016/j.socscimed.2022.102582.

Eigenhuis, Eline, Ruth C. Waumans, Anna D. T. Muntingh, Marjan J. Westerman, Marlinde van Meijel, Neeltje M. Batelaan, and Anton J. L. M. van Balkom. 2021. "Facilitating Factors and Barriers in Help-Seeking Behaviour in Adolescents and Young Adults with Depressive Symptoms: A Qualitative Study." *PLOS ONE* 16 (3): e0247516. https://doi.org/10.1371/journal.pone.0247516.

Eisenberg, Daniel, Ezra Golberstein, and Justin Hunt. 2009. "Mental Health and Academic Success in College." *The B.E. Journal of Economic Analysis & Policy* 9 (1): 40. https://doi.org/10.2202/1935-1682.2191.

Eisenberg, Daniel, Sarah Ketchen Lipson, Justin Heinze, and Sasha Zhou. 2023. *Healthy Minds Study: 2022–2023 Data Report.* Accessed December 6, 2024. https://healthymindsnetwork.org/wp-content/uploads/2023/08/HMS_National-Report-2022-2023_full.pdf.

Eisenberg, Daniel, Sarah Ketchen Lipson, Justin Heinze, and Sasha Zhou. 2024. *Healthy Minds Study 2023–2024 Data Report.* Healthy Minds Network. Accessed December 6, 2024. https://healthymindsnetwork.org/wp-content/uploads/2024/09/HMS_national_report_090924.pdf.

Emerson, Steven, and Brian Duffy. 1990. "Pan Am 103: The German Connection." *New York Times Magazine*, March 18, 1990. https://www.nytimes.com/1990/03/18/magazine/pan-am-103-the-german-connection.html?searchResultPosition=26.

Erdem, Cahit, Eylem Oruç, Cihat Atar, and Hakkı Bağcı. 2023. "The Mediating Effect of Digital Literacy in the Relationship Between Media Literacy and Digital Citizenship." *Education and Information Technologies* 28: 4875–91. https://doi.org/10.1007/s10639-022-11354-4.

Eristi, Bahadir, and Cahit Erdem. 2017. "Development of a Media Literacy Skills Scale." *Contemporary Educational Technology* 8 (3): 249–67. https://doi.org/10.30935/cedtech/6199.

Eshet-Alkalai, Yoram. 2012. "Thinking in the Digital Era: A Revised Model for Digital Literacy." *Issues in Informing Science and Information Technology* 9: 267–76. https://doi.org/10.28945/1621.

Eshet-Alkalai, Yoram, and Yair Amichai-Hamburger. 2004. "Experiments in Digital Literacy." *CyberPsychology & Behavior* 7 (4): 421–29. https://doi.org/10.1089/cpb.2004.7.421.

Feuerstein, Mira. 1999. "Media Literacy in Support of Critical Thinking." *Journal of Educational Media* 24 (1): 43–54. doi:10.1080/1358165990240104.

Flaherty, Colleen. 2023. "Survey: Half of College Students With Mental Health Issues Haven't Accessed Care." *Inside Higher Ed*, May 26, 2023. https://www.insidehighered.com/news/student-success/health-wellness/2023/05/26/gaps-mental-health-care-college-students.

Flannery, Mary Ellen. 2023. "The Mental Health Crisis on College Campuses." *NEA Today*, March 29, 2023. https://www.nea.org/nea-today/all-news-articles/mental-health-crisis-college-campuses.

Fortuna, Karen L., Stephanie Lebby, Pamela Geiger, et al. 2023. "Lived Experience–Led Research Agenda to Address Early Death in People with a Diagnosis of a Serious Mental Illness: A Consensus Statement." *JAMA Network Open* 6, no. 5 (May): e2315479. https://doi.org/10.1001/jamanetworkopen.2023.15479.

Freeman, Becky, Suzette Potente, Vicki Rock, and Justine McIver. 2015. "Social Media Campaigns That Make a Difference: What Can Public Health Learn from the Corporate Sector and Other Social Change Marketers?" *Public Health Research & Practice* 25 (2): e2521517. https://doi.org/10.17061/phrp2521517.

Fresno County Department of Behavioral Health. n.d. "Mental Health Stigma Reduction." Accessed December 13, 2024. https://www.fresnocountyca.gov/Departments/Behavioral-Health/Care-Services/Mental-Health-Stigma-Reduction.

Fresno County Department of Public Health. n.d. *At a Glance: Prescription Opioids 2017 to 2021*. Accessed December 13, 2024. https://www.fresnocountyca.gov/files/assets/county/v/1/public-health/epidemiology-surveillance-and-data-management/other-reports/at-a-glance-prescription-opiods-2017-to-2021.pdf.

Fresno County Sheriff's Office. 2023. *2023 Coroner Unit Statistics*. Accessed December 13, 2024. https://www.fresnosheriff.org/images/pdfs/2023_Coroner_Unit_Statistics_Final.pdf.

Fresno County Suicide Prevention Collaborative. n.d. "Fresno Cares." Accessed December 13, 2024. https://fresnocares.org/.

Fresno State Student Health and Counseling Center. n.d. "Let's Talk." Accessed December 14, 2024. https://studentaffairs.fresnostate.edu/health/counseling/lets-talk.html.

Friesem, Elizaveta, and Yonty Friesem. 2019. "Media Literacy Education through Kuhn's Model of Scientific Revolutions." *Media Education Lab*, March 14, 2019. https://mediaedlab.com/2019/03/14/scientific-revolutions-media-literacy/.

Gagnon Michelle, Bethany L. Gelinas, and Lindsay N. Friesen. 2017. "Mental Health Literacy in Emerging Adults in a University Setting: Distinctions Between Symptom Awareness and Appraisal." *Journal of Adolescent Research* 32 (5): 642–64. https://doi.org/10.1177/0743558415605383.

Gallup. 2023. "US Depression Rates Reach New Highs." *Gallup News*, May 17, 2023. https://news.gallup.com/poll/505745/depression-rates-reach-new-highs.aspx.

Garrido, Sandra, Nikki Millington, Nathan S. Cheers, and Robert J. Boydell. 2019. "What Works and What Doesn't Work? A Systematic Review of Digital Mental Health Interventions for Depression and Anxiety in Young People." *Frontiers in Psychiatry* 10: 759. https://doi.org/10.3389/fpsyt.2019.00759.

Garrido, Sandra, Eliza Oliver, Anthony Chmiel, Barbara Doran, and Katherine Boydell. 2022. "Encouraging Help-Seeking and Engagement in a Mental Health App: What Young People Want." *Frontiers in Digital Health* 4: 1045765. https://doi.org/10.3389/fdgth.2022.1045765.

GBD 2019 Mental Disorders Collaborators. 2022. "Global, Regional, and National Burden of 12 Mental Disorders in 204 Countries and Territories, 1990–2019: A Systematic Analysis for the Global Burden of Disease Study 2019." *The Lancet Psychiatry* 9 (2): 137–50. https://doi.org/10.1016/S2215-0366(21)00395-3.

Goldberg, Marvin E., Keith E. Niedermeier, and Gerald J. Gorn. 2006. "Heightening Adolescent Vigilance Toward Alcohol Advertising to Forestall Alcohol Use." *Journal of Public Policy & Marketing* 25 (2): 147–59. https://doi.org/10.1509/jppm.25.2.147.

Goodwin, John, and Laura Behan. 2023. "Does Media Content Have an Impact on Help-Seeking Behaviors for Mental Illness? A Systematic Review." *Mental Health Review Journal* 28 (3): 283–302. https://doi.org/10.1108/MHRJ-06-2022-0038.

Greenwood, Hannah, Natalia Krzyzaniak, Ruwani Peiris, Justin Clark, Anna Mae Scott, Magnolia Cardona, Rebecca Griffith, and Paul Glasziou. 2022. "Telehealth Versus Face-to-face Psychotherapy for Less Common Mental Health Conditions: Systematic Review and Meta-analysis of Randomized Controlled Trials." *JMIR Mental Health* 9 (3): e31780. https://doi.org/10.2196/31780.

Gretter, Sarah, and Aman Yadav. 2018. "What Do Preservice Teachers Think about Teaching Media Literacy? An Exploratory Study Using the Theory of Planned Behavior." *Journal of Media Literacy Education* 10 (1). https://digitalcommons.uri.edu/jmle/vol10/iss1/6/.

Guess, Andrew M., Michael Lerner, Benjamin Lyons, Jacob M. Montgomery, Brendan Nyhan, Jason Reifler, and Neelanjan Sircar. 2020. "A Digital Media Literacy Intervention Increases Discernment Between Mainstream and False News in the United States and India." *Princeton School of Public and International Affairs* 117 (27): 15536–45. https://collaborate.princeton.edu/en/publications/a-digital-media-literacy-intervention-increases-discernment-betwe.

Gupta, Monica, Amita Jassi, and Georgina Krebs. 2023. "The Association Between Social Media Use and Body Dysmorphic Symptoms in Young People." *Frontiers in Psychology* 14: 1231801. https://doi.org/10.3389/fpsyg.2023.1231801.

Haidt, Jonathan. 2023. "Social Media Is a Major Cause of the Mental Illness Epidemic in Teen Girls. Here's the Evidence." *After Babel* (blog), February 22, 2023. https://www.afterbabel.com/p/social-media-mental-illness-epidemic.

Haidt, Jonathan. 2024. *How Social Media is Harming Young Minds.* YouTube video, 23:47. Posted December 15, 2024. https://www.youtube.com/watch?v=csubiPlvFWk.

Hancock, Jeff, Sunny Xun Liu, Mufan Luo, and Hannah Mieczkowski. 2022. "Psychological Well-Being and Social Media Use: A Meta-Analysis of Associations between Social Media Use and Depression, Anxiety, Loneliness, Eudaimonic, Hedonic, and Social Well-Being." *SSRN Electronic Journal*, April 15, 2022. https://papers.ssrn.com/sol3/papers.cfm?abstract_id=4053961.

Haraldsson, Johanna, Ronnie Pingel, Lena Nordgren, Linus Johnsson, Per Kristiansson, and Ylva Tindberg. 2022. "Confidentiality Matters! Adolescent Males' Views of Primary Care in Relation to Psychosocial Health: A Structural Equation Modelling Approach." *Scandinavian Journal of Primary Health Care* 40 (4): 492–501. https://doi.org/10.1080/02813432.2022.2144999.

Hardey, Mariann, and Rowland Atkinson. 2019. "Disconnected: Non-Users of Information Communication Technologies." *Sociological Research Online* 23 (3): 621–38. https://doi.org/10.1177/1360780418764736.

Harrer, Mathias, Sophia H. Adam, Harald Baumeister, Pim Cuijpers, Eirini Karyotaki, Randy P. Auerbach, Ronald C. Kessler, Ronny Bruffaerts, Matthias Berking, and David D. Ebert. 2019. "Internet Interventions for Mental Health in University Students: A Systematic Review and Meta-Analysis." *International Journal of Methods in Psychiatric Research* 28 (2): e1759. https://doi.org/10.1002/mpr.1759.

Harvard Medical School/Children's Hospital Digital Wellness Lab. n.d. "Digital Wellness Lab." Accessed December 21, 2024. https://digitalwellnesslab.org.

Hayes, Daniel, Rosie Mansfield, Carla Mason, Joao Santos, Anna Moore, Jan Boehnke, Emma Ashworth, Bettina Moltrecht, Neil Humphrey, Paul Stallard, Praveetha Patalay, and Jessica Deighton. 2024. "The Impact of Universal, School-Based, Interventions on Help-Seeking in Children and Young People: A Systematic Literature Review." *European Child & Adolescent Psychiatry* 33 (9): 2911–28. https://doi.org/10.1007/s00787-022-02135-y.

Healthy Fresno County. n.d. *Healthy Fresno County Community Dashboard: Mental Health.* Accessed December 13, 2024. https://www.healthyfresnocountydata.org/index.php?module=indicators&controller=index&action=dashboard&alias=mentalhealth.

Healthy Minds Network. 2023. *Healthy Minds Study: 2022-2023 Data Report.* Accessed December 3, 2024. https://healthymindsnetwork.org/wp-content/uploads/2023/08/HMS_National-Report-2022-2023_full.pdf.

Hellström, Lisa, and Linda Beckman. 2021. "Life Challenges and Barriers to Help Seeking: Adolescents' and Young Adults' Voices of Mental Health." *International Journal of Environmental Research and Public Health* 18 (24): 13101. https://doi.org/10.3390/ijerph182413101.

Hensel, Andrew. 2022. "Senate Bill Seeks to Add Media Literacy to High School Curriculum." *Patch*, February 15, 2022. https://patch.com/illinois/chicago/senate-bill-seeks-add-media-literacy-high-school-curriculum#google_vignette.

Hern, Alex. 2014. "Facebook Deliberately Made People Sad. This Ought to Be the Final Straw." *The Guardian*, June 30, 2014. https://www.theguardian.com/commentisfree/2014/jun/30/facebook-sad-manipulating-emotions-socially-responsible-company.

Hines, Eric, Tracee L. Perryman, and Donald L. Perryman. *Culturally Responsive Mental Health Services: Engaging Diverse Populations.* Center of Hope Family Services, 2023. https://cohfs.org/sites/default/files/inline-files/Culturally%20Responsive%20Mental%20Health%20Services%20%28FINAL%20FiNAL%209-14-23%29.pdf.

Higdon, Nolan. 2022. "The Critical Effect: Exploring the Influence of Critical Media Literacy Pedagogy on College Students' Social Media Behaviors and Attitudes." *Journal of Media Literacy Education* 14 (1): 1–13. https://doi.org/10.23860/JMLE-2022-14-1-1.

Hobbs, Renee. 1994. "Pedagogical Issues in US Media Education." *Communication Yearbook* 17: 453–66. https://doi.org/10.1080/23808985.1994.11678897.

Hobbs, Renee. 1998. *The Seven Great Debates in the Media Literacy Movement.* National Telemedia Council. https://eric.ed.gov/?id=ED439454.

Hobbs, Renee. 2017. "Measuring the Digital and Media Literacy Competencies of Children and Teens." In *Cognitive Development in Digital Contexts*, edited by Fran C. Blumberg and Patricia J. Brooks. Academic Press.

Hobbs, Renee. 2005. "The State of Media Literacy Education." *Journal of Communication* 55 (4): 865–871. https://doi.org/10.1111/j.1460-2466.2005.tb03027.x.

Hobbs, Renee. 2021. *Media Literacy in Action: Questioning the Media*, 2nd ed. Rowman & Littlefield.

Hobbs, Renee, and Amy Jensen. 2009. "The Past, Present, and Future of Media Literacy Education." *Journal of Media Literacy Education* 1 (1): 1–11. https://digitalcommons.uri.edu/jmle/vol1/iss1/1.

Hochbaum, Godfrey M. 1958. *Public Participation in Medical Screening Programs: A Socio-psychological Study*. US Government Printing Office.

Hossain, Imran, and A.K.M. Mahmudul Haque. 2023. "The Role of Social Media in Spreading Rumors in Bangladesh During COVID-19 Pandemic." *SSRN Electronic Journal*. http://ijeais.org/wp-content/uploads/2023/1/IJAMR230133.pdf.

Hughes, Karen, Mark A. Bellis, Katherine A. Hardcastle, Dinesh Sethi, Alexander Butchart, and Christopher Mikton. 2017. "The Effect of Multiple Adverse Childhood Experiences on Health: A Systematic Review and Meta-Analysis." *The Lancet Public Health* 2 (8): e356–66. https://doi.org/10.1016/S2468-2667(17)30118-4.

Hunter, Ruth F., Kayla de la Haye, Jennifer M. Murray, Jennifer Badham, Thomas W. Valente, Mike Clarke, and Frank Kee. 2019. "Social Network Interventions for Health Behaviours and Outcomes: A Systematic Review and Meta-Analysis." *PLoS Medicine* 16 (9): e1002890. https://doi.org/10.1371/journal.pmed.1002890.

Ibarra-Mejia, Gabriel, Mark Lusk, and Emre Umucu. 2023. "Mental Health Among College Students During the COVID-19 Pandemic at a Hispanic-Serving Institution." *Health Promotion Practice* 24 (3): 419–29. https://doi.org/10.1177/15248399221092750.

Ibrahim, Rasha Kadri, Saher Al Sabbah, Muhammed Al-Jarrah, John Senior, Jehad Ali Almomani, Amani Darwish, Faisal Albannay, and Ahmad Al Naimat. 2024. "The Mediating Effect of Digital Literacy and Self-Regulation on the Relationship between Emotional Intelligence and Academic Stress among University Students: A Cross-Sectional Study." *BMC Medical Education* 24: 739. https://doi.org/10.1186/s12909-024-06279-0.

Ikeda, Shinnosuke. 2023. "The More Emotional Words You Know, the Higher Your Mental Health." *Scandinavian Journal of Psychology* 64 (6): 705–9. https://doi.org/10.1111/sjop.12928.

Illinois General Assembly. 2021a. "House Roll Call, House Bill 234: SCH CD-Media Literacy, Third Reading, Passed." *Illinois General Assembly*, April 20, 2021. https://www.ilga.gov/legislation/votehistory/102/house/10200HB0234_04202021_002000T.pdf.

Illinois General Assembly. 2021b. *Public Act 102-0055*, Sec. 27-20.08. https://www.ilga.gov/Legislation/publicacts/view/102-0055.

International Accreditation of Counseling Services. n.d. "Frequently Asked Questions." Accessed December 14, 2024. https://iacsinc.org/faq.

Irving, Lyn M., Jennifer DuPen, and Susan Berel. 1998. "A Media Literacy Program for High School Females." *Eating Disorders: The Journal of Treatment & Prevention* 6 (2): 119–32. https://doi.org/10.1080/10640269808251248.

Jackson, Stanley W. 2024. "Melancholia and Depression: From Hippocrates to Modern Times." In *The Oxford Handbook of the History of Medicine*, edited by Mark Jackson, 121–45. Oxford University Press. https://academic.oup.com/edited-volume/41353/chapter-abstract/352517403.

Jagosh, Justin, Corey McAuliffe, Liza McGuinness, Trevor Goodyear, Rebecca Haines-Saah, Zachary Daly, Tanya Halsall, Taylor G. Hill, Tyesa Kruz, Joan Wandolo, Tasneet Suri, and Emily Jenkins. 2024. "Identifying Mechanisms of Youth Mental Health Promotion: A Realist Evaluation of the Agenda Gap Programme." *PLOS Mental Health* 1 (1): e0000068. https://doi.org/10.1371/journal.pmen.0000068.

Jardine, Jacinta, Robert Bowman, and Gavin Doherty. 2022. "Digital Interventions to Enhance Readiness for Psychological Therapy: Scoping Review." *Journal of Medical Internet Research* 24 (8): e37851. https://doi.org/10.2196/37851.

Jaycox, Lisa H., Eric R. Murphy, Julia L. Zehr, Jane L. Pearson, and Shelli Avenevoli. 2023. "Social Media and Suicide Risk in Youth." *JAMA Network Open* 6 (9): e2825340. https://doi.org/10.1001/jamanetworkopen.2023.25340.

Jellestad, Lena, Nicolà A. Vital, Jolanda Malamud, Jan Taeymans, and Christoph Mueller-Pfeiffer. 2021. "Functional Impairment in Posttraumatic Stress Disorder: A Systematic Review and Meta-Analysis." *Journal of Psychiatric Research* 140: 202–16. https://doi.org/10.1016/j.jpsychires.2021.02.015.

Jeong, Se-Hoon, Nicholas D. H. Cho, and Kyungboon Hwang. 2012. "Media Literacy Interventions: A Meta-Analytic Review." *Journal of Communication* 62 (3): 454–72. https://doi.org/10.1111/j.1460-2466.2012.01643.x.

Jiayuan, Zhou, Lina Ma, and Lihong Yang. 2025. "Problematic Media Use, Mental Health Literacy, and Their Interaction in Depression among Nursing Students." *BMC Nursing* 24: 199. https://doi.org/10.1186/s12912-025-02827-1.

Johns, David J., Tessa E. Langley, and Sarah Lewis. 2017. "Use of Social Media for the Delivery of Health Promotion on Smoking, Nutrition, and Physical Activity: A Systematic Review." *The Lancet* 390: S49. https://doi.org/10.1016/S0140-6736(17)32984-7.

Johnson, Jemimah A., Janhavi Devdutt, Seema Mehrotra, Poornima Bhola, Paulomi Sudhir, and Amit Sharma. 2020. "Barriers to Professional Help-Seeking for Distress and Potential Utility of a Mental Health App Components: Stakeholder Perspectives." *Cureus* 12 (2): e7128. https://doi.org/10.7759/cureus.7128.

Johnson, Jemimah A., Prachi Sanghvi, and Seema Mehrotra. 2021. "Technology-Based Interventions to Improve Help-Seeking for Mental Health Concerns: A Systematic Review." *Indian Journal of Psychological Medicine* 44 (4): 332–40. https://doi.org/10.1177/02537176211034578.

Johnson, Sharon. 2024. "Media Literacy Becomes a State Issue." *The Progressive*, June 3, 2024. https://progressive.org/magazine/media-literacy-becomes-a-state-issue-johnson-20240603/.

Johnston, David. 1991. "Flight 103: A Solution Assembled From Fragments and Debris." *New York Times*, November 15, 1991. https://www.nytimes.com/1991/11/15/world/flight-103-a-solution-assembled-from-fragments-and-debris.html?searchResultPosition=35.

Jones, Carolyn. 2023. "Recognizing Fake News Now a Required Subject in California Schools." *CalMatters*, November 10, 2023. https://calmatters.org/education/k-12-education/2023/11/fake-news-california-school/.

Jones, Sandra C., Lisa Kervin, and Chloe Hindmarsh. 2015. "Effectiveness of Alcohol Media Literacy Programmes: A Systematic Literature Review." *Health Education Research* 30 (3): 449–65. https://doi.org/10.1093/her/cyv017.

Jorm, Anthony F. 2012. "Mental Health Literacy: Empowering the Community to Take Action for Better Mental Health." *American Psychologist* 67 (3): 231–43. https://doi.org/10.1037/a0025957.

Jorm, Anthony F., Ailsa E. Korten, Patricia A. Jacomb, Helen Christensen, Bryan Rodgers, and Penelope Pollitt. 1997. "Mental Health Literacy: A Survey of the Public's Ability to Recognise Mental Disorders and Their Beliefs about the Effectiveness of Treatment." *Medical Journal of Australia* 166 (4): 182–6. https://www.mja.com.au/journal/1997/166/4/mental-health-literacy-survey-publics-ability-recognise-mental-disorders-and.

Kellner, Douglas, and Jeff Share. 2005. "Toward Critical Media Literacy: Core Concepts, Debates, Organizations, and Policy." *Discourse: Studies in the Cultural Politics of Education* 26 (3): 369–86. https://doi.org/10.1080/01596300500200169.

Kessler, Ronald C., G. Paul Amminger, Sergio Aguilar-Gaxiola, Jordi Alonso, Sing Lee, and T. Bedirhan Üstün. 2007. "Age of Onset of Mental Disorders: A Review of Recent Literature." *Current Opinion in Psychiatry* 20 (4): 359–64. https://doi.org/10.1097/YCO.0b013e32816ebc8c.

Knaus, Thomas. 2022. "Making in Media Education: An Activity-Oriented Approach to Digital Literacy." *Journal of Media Literacy Education* 14 (3): 53–65. https://digitalcommons.uri.edu/jmle/vol14/iss3/5.

Knettel, Brandon A., Pranav Ganapathy, and Conner Rougier-Chapman. 2023. "Examining Factors Associated with Mental Health Stigma and Attitudes Toward Help-Seeking among International College Students during the COVID-19 Pandemic." *PLOS Mental Health* 2 (9): e0000063. https://doi.org/10.1371/journal.pmen.0000063.

Kosic, Marianna. 2018. "Media Literacy and for the Net Generation." *International Journal of Emotional Education* 10 (1): 68–88. https://files.eric.ed.gov/fulltext/EJ1177650.pdf.

Kramer, Adam D. I., Jamie E. Guillory, and Jeffrey T. Hancock. 2014. "Experimental Evidence of Massive-Scale Emotional Contagion through Social Networks." *Proceedings of the National Academy of Sciences of the United States of America* 111 (24): 8788–90. https://doi.org/10.1073/pnas.1320040111.

Kross, Ethan, Philippe Verduyn, Gal Sheppes, Cory K. Costello, John Jonides, and Oscar Ybarra. 2021. "Social Media and Well-Being: Pitfalls, Progress, and Next Steps." *Trends in Cognitive Sciences* 25 (1): 55–66. https://doi.org/10.1016/j.tics.2020.10.005.

Kurz, Martina, Jenny Rosendahl, Johanna Rodeck, Julia Muehleck, and Uwe Berger. 2022. "School-Based Interventions Improve Body Image and Media Literacy in Youth: A Systematic Review and Meta-Analysis." *The Journal of Primary Prevention* 43 (1): 51–77. https://doi.org/10.1007/s10935-021-00660-1.

Langreo, Lauraine. 2022. "A Media Literacy Requirement That Starts in Kindergarten? New Jersey May Start the Trend." *Education Week*, November 23, 2022. https://www.edweek.org/teaching-learning/a-media-literacy-requirement-that-starts-in-kindergarten-new-jersey-may-start-the-trend/2022/11.

Langreo, Lauraine. 2023. "What Teachers Need to Know About AI, But Don't: Students Must Be Critical AI Users. 3 Steps for Teachers to Prepare." *Education Week*, August 31, 2023. https://www.edweek.org/technology/what-teachers-need-to-know-about-ai-but-dont/2023/08.

Latha, K., K. S. Meena, M. R. Pravitha, Madhuporna Dasgupta, and S. K. Chaturvedi. 2020. "Effective Use of Social Media Platforms for Promotion of Mental Health Awareness." *Journal of Education and Health Promotion* 9: 124. Wolters Kluwer - Medknow. https://jehp.mui.ac.ir/article_29084_9f7e82b8f2ac927f6766d55fff02843a.pdf.

Leech, Teghan, Diana Dorstyn, Amanda Taylor, and Wenjing Li. 2021. "Mental Health Apps for Adolescents and Young Adults: A Systematic Review of Randomised Controlled Trials." *Children and Youth Services Review* 127: 106073. https://doi.org/10.1016/j.childyouth.2021.106073.

Lee, John H., and Emma C. Smith. 2023. "Managing Information Overload in Healthcare: Challenges and Solutions in the Digital Age." *Personal and Ubiquitous Computing* 27 (4): 523–36. https://doi.org/10.1007/s00779-023-01710-7.

Legislative Analyst's Office. 2021. *Overview of Mental Health Services for College Students*. December 10, 2021. https://lao.ca.gov/Publications/Report/4481.

Lehtimaki, Susanna, Jana Martic, Brian Wahl, Katherine T. Foster, and Nina Schwalbe. 2021. "Evidence on Digital Mental Health Interventions for Adolescents and Young People: Systematic Overview." *JMIR Mental Health* 8 (4): e25847. https://doi.org/10.2196/25847.

Levin-Zamir, Diane, and Isabella Bertschi. (2018). "Media Health Literacy, eHealth Literacy and the Role of the Social Environments in Context." *International Journal of Environmental Research and Public Health* 15: 1643–55. https://doi.org/10.3390/ijerph15081643.

Lewis, Justin, and Sut Jhally. 1998. "The Struggle Over Media Literacy." *Journal of Communication* 48 (1): 109–120. https://doi.org/10.1111/j.1460-2466.1998.tb02741.x.

Lipson, Sarah Ketchen, Alejandro Heiman, Kristina C. Elmer, Sasha K. Klingensmith, and Daniel Eisenberg. 2018. "Mental Health Disparities Among College Students of Color." *Journal of Adolescent Health* 63 (3): 348–56. https://doi.org/10.1016/j.jadohealth.2018.04.014.

Lipson, Sarah Ketchen, Megan V. Phillips, Nathan Winquist, Daniel Eisenberg, and Emily G. Lattie. 2021. "Mental Health Conditions Among Community College Students: A National Study of Prevalence and Use of Treatment Services." *Psychiatric Services* 72 (10): 1126–33. https://doi.org/10.1176/appi.ps.202000437.

Lipson, Sarah Ketchen, Sasha Zhou, Sara Abelson, Justin Heinze, Matthew Jirsa, Jasmine Morigney, Akilah Patterson, Meghna Singh, and Daniel Eisenberg. 2022. "Trends in College Student Mental Health and Help-Seeking by Race/Ethnicity: Findings from the National Healthy Minds Study, 2013–2021." *Journal of Affective Disorders* 306: 138–47. https://doi.org/10.1016/j.jad.2022.03.038.

Lin, Tzu-Bin, Jin Li, Fang Deng, and Lung-Hsiang Lee. 2013. "Understanding New Media Literacy: An Explorative Theoretical Framework." *Educational Technology & Society* 16 (4): 160–70. https://www.jstor.org/stable/jeductechsoci.16.4.160.

Literat, Ioana, Yoo Kyung Chang, Joseph Eisman, and Jonathan Gardner. 2021. "LAMBOOZLED!: The Design and Development of a Game-Based Approach to News Literacy Education." *Journal of Media Literacy Education* 13 (1): 56–66. https://doi.org/10.23860/JMLE-2021-13-1-5.

Liu, Jiaying, and Yan Zhang. 2024. "Understanding and Facilitating Mental Health Help-Seeking of Young Adults: A Socio-technical Ecosystem Framework." *arXiv Preprint*. https://arxiv.org/abs/2401.08994v1.

Liu, Jiaying, and Yan Zhang. 2025. "When I Lost It, They Dragged Me Out: How Care Encounters Empower Marginalized Young Adults' Mental Health Care-Seeking." *arXiv Preprint*, February 16, 2025. https://arxiv.org/abs/2502.11277.

Livingstone, Sonia. 2004. "Media Literacy and the Challenge of New Information and Communication Technologies." *The Communication Review* 7 (1): 3–14. https://www.tandfonline.com/doi/abs/10.1080/10714420490280152.

Lowenstein, Peter. 1997. "Call Libya's Bluff on a Pan Am 103 Trial." *New York Times*, November 3, 1997. https://www.nytimes.com/1997/11/03/opinion/l-call-libya-s-bluff-on-a-pan-am-103-trial-902900.html?searchResultPosition=25.

Manca, Stefania, Stefania Bocconi, and Benjamin Gleason. 2021. "'Think Globally, Act Locally': A Glocal Approach to the Development of Social Media Literacy." *Computers & Education* 160: 104025. https://doi.org/10.1016/j.compedu.2020.104025.

Martin, Rachel. 2022. "Illinois Now Requires Media Literacy Instruction in Its High School Curriculum." *NPR*, September 14, 2022. https://www.npr.org/2022/09/14/1122895362/illinois-now-requires-media-literacy-instruction-in-its-high-school-curriculum.

Martin, Saleen. 2023. "Recognizing Fake News: Media Literacy Now Required Subject in California Schools." *USA Today*, November 21, 2023. https://www.usatoday.com/story/news/education/2023/11/21/fake-news-california-schools-media-literacy/71664379007/.

McGuire, William J. 1961. "The Effectiveness of Supportive and Refutational Defenses in Immunizing and Restoring Beliefs Against Persuasion." *Sociometry* 24: 184–97. https://doi.org/10.2307/2786067.

McKenzie, Sarah K., Sunny Collings, Gabrielle Jenkin, and Jo River. 2018. "Masculinity, Social Connectedness, and Mental Health: Men's Diverse Patterns of Practice." *American Journal of Men's Health* 12 (1): 124–34. https://doi.org/10.1177/1557988317745913.

McLean, Sarah, Eleanor Wertheim, Jessica Masters, and Susan Paxton. 2017. "A Pilot Evaluation of a Social Media Literacy Intervention to Reduce Risk Factors for Eating Disorders." *International Journal of Eating Disorders* 50 (7): 847–51. https://doi.org/10.1002/eat.22708.

McNeill, Erin, and Michelle Carter. 2024. "Tips for Teaching Media Literacy in Skills-Based Health Education." *SHAPE America Blog*, July 25, 2024. https://blog.shapeamerica.org/2024/07/tips-for-teaching-media-literacy-in-skills-based-health-education/.

McNelly, Tracy A., and Jessica Harvey. 2021. "Media Literacy Instruction in Today's Classrooms: A Study of Teachers' Knowledge, Confidence, and Integration." *Journal of Media Literacy Education* 13 (1). https://digitalcommons.uri.edu/jmle/vol13/iss1/10/.

Meadley, Abigail, Debra Rickwood, and Amelia Ishikawa. 2024. "Young Adults' Perceptions of the Role of Self-Reliance and Trust on Help Seeking for Mental Health Problems." *Youth* 4 (4): 1726–38. https://doi.org/10.3390/youth4040109.

Media Literacy Now. n.d. "Resource Library." Accessed December 19, 2024. https://medialiteracynow.org/resource-library/.

Media Literacy Now. 2022. "National Survey Finds Most US Adults Have Not Had Media Literacy Education in High School." Accessed December 19, 2024. https://medialiteracynow.org/nationalsurvey2022/.

Media Literacy Now. 2023. *Media Literacy Now Policy Report 2023*, February 2024. https://medialiteracynow.org/wp-content/uploads/2024/02/MediaLiteracyNowPolicyReport2023_publishedFeb2024b.pdf.

Media Literacy Now. 2024. "Current Policy." *Media Literacy Now*. Accessed November 30. https://medialiteracynow.org/impact/current-policy/.

Medill Local News Initiative. 2023. "More Than Half of US Counties Have No Access or Very Limited Access to Local News." *Medill School of Journalism, Northwestern University*. Accessed December 3, 2024. https://www.medill.northwestern.edu/news/2023/more-than-half-of-us-counties-have-no-access-or-very-limited-access-to-local-news.html.

Micali, Nadia, Maria G. Martini, Jennifer J. Thomas, Kamryn T. Eddy, Roshni Kothari, Elizabeth Russell, Cynthia M. Bulik, and Janet Treasure. 2017. "Lifetime and 12-Month Prevalence of Eating Disorders amongst Women in Mid-Life: A Population-Based Study of Diagnoses and Risk Factors." *BMC Medicine* 15 (1): 1–12. https://doi.org/10.1186/s12916-016-0766-4.

Michel, Chantal, Nina Schnyder, Stefanie J. Schmidt, Nicola Groth, Benno G. Schimmelmann, and Frauke Schultze-Lutter. 2021. "Functioning Mediates Help-Seeking for Mental Problems in the General Population." *European Psychiatry* 64 (1): e65. https://doi.org/10.1192/j.eurpsy.2021.65.

Michel, Christina, Nathalie Schnyder, Sarah J. Schmidt, Nadine Groth, and Frauke Schultze-Lutter. 2018. "Functioning Mediates Help-Seeking for Mental Problems in the General Population." *European Psychiatry* 53: 9–17. https://doi.org/10.1016/j.eurpsy.2018.05.001.

Mickle, Tripp. 2021. "YouTube's Search Algorithm Directs Viewers to False and Sexualized Videos, Study Finds." *Wall Street Journal*, July 6, 2021. https://www.wsj.com/articles/youtubes-search-algorithm-directs-viewers-to-false-and-sexualized-videos-study-finds-11625644803.

Migration Policy Institute. n.d. "Profile of the Unauthorized Population: Fresno County, CA." Accessed December 14, 2024. https://www.migrationpolicy.org/data/unauthorized-immigrant-population/county/6019.

Mihailidis, Paul, and Benjamin Thevenin. 2013. "Media Literacy as a Core Competency for Engaged Citizenship in Participatory Democracy." *American Behavioral Scientist* 57 (11): 1611–22. https://doi.org/10.1177/0002764213489015.

Mihailidis, Paul, and Benjamin Thevenin. 2017. "Media Literacy as a Core Competency for Engaged Citizenship in Participatory Democracy." *Journal of Media Literacy Education* 9 (1): 79–98. https://digitalcommons.uri.edu/jmle/vol9/iss1/6/.

Milne-Ives, Madison, Emma Selby, Becky Inkster, Ching Lam, and Edward Meinert. 2022. "Artificial Intelligence and Machine Learning in Mobile Apps for Mental Health: A Scoping Review." *PLOS Digital Health* 1 (8): e0000079. https://doi.org/10.1371/journal.pdig.0000079.

Mitchell, Caroline, Brian McMillan, and Teresa Hagan. 2017. "Mental Health Help Seeking in Young Adults." *British Journal of General Practice* 67 (654): 8–9. https://doi.org/10.3399/bjgp17X688453.

Modi, Hemangi, Kendal Orgera, and Atul Grover. 2022. *Barriers to Mental Health Care*. AAMC Research and Action Institute, Washington D.C., October 10, 2022. https://www.aamc.org/media/83701/download.

Molander, Olof, Josefin Särnholm, Anna-Clara Hollander, and Nitya Jayaram-Lindström. 2024. "Mind the Gap: Scaling-Up Access to Culturally Adapted Mental Health Treatments for Minority Populations." *BMC Global and Public Health* 2: 61. https://doi.org/10.1186/s44263-024-00092-z.

Moss, Lolita, and Lisa Fedina. 2022. "Centering Media Literacy and Cultural Tailoring: A Scoping Review of Interventions Used to Address Black Adolescent Intimate Partner Violence." *Trauma, Violence, & Abuse* 24 (4): 2181–95. https://doi.org/10.1177/15248380221090493.

Mrazek, A. J., M. D. Mrazek, C. M. Cherolini, J. N. Cloughesy, D. J. Cynman, L. J. Gougis, A. P. Landry, J. V. Reese, and J. W. Schooler. 2019. "The Future of Mindfulness Training Is Digital, and the Future Is Now." *Current Opinion in Psychology* 28: 81–6. https://doi.org/10.1016/j.copsyc.2018.11.012.

Murphy, Mary C., Maithreyi Gopalan, Evelyn R. Carter, Katherine T. U. Emerson, Bette L. Bottoms, and Gregory M. Walton. 2020. "A Customized Belonging Intervention Improves Retention of Socially Disadvantaged Students at a Broad-Access University." *Science Advances* 6 (29): eaba4677. https://doi.org/10.1126/sciadv.aba4677.

Murthy, Vivek H. 2024. "Surgeon General: Why I'm Calling for a Warning Label on Social Media Platforms." *The New York Times*, June 17, 2024. https://www.nytimes.com/2024/06/17/opinion/social-media-health-warning.html.

Nagengast, Larry. 2023. "Delaware Takes the Lead on Teaching Media Literacy." *Delaware Public Media*, August 25, 2023. https://www.delawarepublic.org/show/the-green/2023-08-25/delaware-takes-the-lead-on-teaching-media-literacy.

National Academies of Sciences, Engineering, and Medicine. 2023. "To Minimize Harms and Maximize Benefits of Social Media to Adolescent Health, New Report Recommends Setting Industrywide Standards, New Protections Against Harassment." *National Academies News*, December 2023. https://www.nationalacademies.org/news/2023/12/to-minimize-harms-and-maximize-benefits-of-social-media-to-adolescent-health-new-report-recommends-setting-industrywide-standards-new-protections-against-harassment.

National Alliance on Mental Illness. n.d. "LGBTQ+." Accessed December 14, 2024. https://www.nami.org/your-journey/identity-and-cultural-dimensions/lgbtq/.

National Association for Media Literacy Education (NAMLE). n.d.a. "Media Literacy Defined." Accessed January 2, 2025. https://namle.org/resources/media-literacy-defined/.

National Association for Media Literacy Education (NAMLE). n.d.b. "Media Literacy Resources." Accessed December 19, 2024. https://namle.net/resources/.

National Association for Media Literacy Education. 2007. "Core Principles of Media Literacy Education in the United States." Accessed June 23, 2025. http://www.amlainfo.org/uploads/r4/cE/r4cEZukacxNYaFFxlMONdQ/NAMLE-CPMLE-w-questions.pdf.

National Center for Education Statistics. 2024. "Public School Enrollment." *Condition of Education.* Accessed November 30. https://nces.ed.gov/programs/coe/indicator/cga/public-school-enrollment.

National Institute of Mental Health. 2024. "Major Depression." Accessed December 1, 2024. https://www.nimh.nih.gov/health/statistics/major-depression.

Nazari, Abouzar, Gholamreza Garmaroudi, and Marzie Rabiei. 2024. "A Systematic Review: Increasing Mental Health Literacy in Students through 'The Guide.'" *Discover Psychology* 4: 96. https://doi.org/10.1007/s44202-024-00219-1.

NBC New York Staff. 2024. "Generation Text: See the Full NBC Survey Results as Principals Reveal Concern about Phones in Schools." *NBC New York*, December 14, 2024. https://www.nbcnewyork.com/news/local/generation-text-see-the-full-nbc-survey-results-as-principals-reveal-concern-about-phones-in-schools/5645963/.

Nelson, Tamara, Naysha N. Shahid, and Esteban V. Cardemil. 2020. "Do I Really Need to Go and See Somebody? Black Women's Perceptions of Help-Seeking for Depression." *Journal of Black Psychology* 46 (4): 263–85. https://doi.org/10.1177/0095798420931644.

New Hampshire Department of Education. n.d. "Mental Health and Academic Achievement." Accessed January 2, 2025. https://www.education.nh.gov/sites/g/files/ehbemt326/files/inline-documents/mental_health_and_academic_achievement.pdf.

New Jersey Legislature. 2023. *Bill S588 ScsAcaAca (SCS/2R), Session 2022–2023: Directs DOE to Develop New Jersey Student Learning Standards in Information Literacy.* New Jersey Legislature. https://www.njleg.state.nj.us/bill-search/2022/S588.

New Mexico Public Education Department. 2024. "Digital Citizenship." *New Mexico Public Education Department.* Accessed November 30. https://webnew.ped.state.nm.us/bureaus/digital-equity/digital-citizenship/.

News Literacy Project. 2024. *News Literacy in America: A Survey of Teen Information Attitudes, Habits, and Skills (2024)*. October 2024. https://newslit.org/wp-content/uploads/2024/10/NLP-Teen-Survey-Report-2024.pdf.

Nguyen, Minh-Hoang, Xuan-Thanh Nguyen, Thi-Hai-Ha Tran, Thu-Trang Nguyen, Duc-Khanh Tran, and Van-Tam Nguyen. 2021. "Alice in Suicideland: Exploring the Suicidal Ideation Mechanism through the Sense of Connectedness and Help-Seeking Behaviors." *International Journal of Environmental Research and Public Health* 18 (7): 3681. https://doi.org/10.3390/ijerph18073681.

Niederkrotenthaler, Thomas, Daniel J. Reidenberg, Benedikt Till, and Madelyn S. Gould. 2014. "Increasing Help-Seeking and Referrals for Individuals at Risk for Suicide by Decreasing Stigma: The Role of Mass Media." *American Journal of Preventive Medicine* 47 (3 Suppl 2): S235–43. https://doi.org/10.1016/j.amepre.2014.06.010.

Ni Shuilleabhain, Niamh, Emma Rich, and Simone Fullagar. 2021. "Rethinking Digital Media Literacy to Address Body Dissatisfaction in Schools: Lessons from Feminist New Materialisms." *New Media & Society* 25 (12): 3247–65. https://doi.org/10.1177/14614448211041715.

Noh, Dabok, and Hyunlye Kim. 2023. "Effectiveness of Online Interventions for the Universal and Selective Prevention of Mental Health Problems Among Adolescents: A Systematic Review and Meta-Analysis." *Prevention Science* 24 (1): 353–64. https://doi.org/10.1007/s11121-022-01443-8.

Nutbeam, Don. 2008. "The Evolving Concept of Health Literacy." *Social Science & Medicine* 67 (12): 2072–8. https://doi.org/10.1016/j.socscimed.2008.09.050.

Office of the Governor. 2023. "Governor Murphy Signs First-in-the-Nation Legislation Requiring K-12 Instruction on Information Literacy." *State of New Jersey*, January 4, 2023. https://www.nj.gov/governor/news/news/562022/20230104b.shtml#:~:text=%E2%80%9COur%20democracy%20remains%20under%20sustained,to%20identify%20fact%20from%20fiction.

Ohanian, Lee. 2023. "New California Law Requires 'Fake News' Classes for K–12 Students." *Hoover Institution*, November 14, 2023. https://www.hoover.org/research/new-california-law-requires-fake-news-classes-k-12-students.

Okolo, Chioma Anthonia, Rawlings Chidi, Oloruntoba Babawarun, Jeremiah Olawumi Arowoogun, and Adekunle Oyeyemi Adeniyi. 2024. "Data-Driven Approaches to Bridging the Gap in Health Communication Disparities: A Systematic Review." *World Journal of Advanced Research and Reviews* 21 (2): 1435–45. https://doi.org/10.30574/wjarr.2024.21.2.0591.

O'Neill, Alisha, Emily Stapley, Ishba Rehman, and Neil Humphrey. 2023. "Adolescent Help-Seeking: An Exploration of Associations with Perceived Cause of Emotional Distress." *Frontiers in Psychology* 14: 1057843. https://doi.org/10.3389/fpsyg.2023.1057843.

O'Reilly, Michelle, Nisha Dogra, Jason Hughes, Paul Reilly, Riya George, and Natasha Whiteman. 2019. "Potential of Social Media in Promoting Mental Health in Adolescents." *Health Promotion International* 34 (5): 981–91. https://doi.org/10.1093/heapro/day056.

Osborn, T. G., S. Li, R. Saunders, and P. Fonagy. 2022. "University Students' Use of Mental Health Services: A Systematic Review and Meta-Analysis." *BMC Psychiatry* 22: 753. https://doi.org/10.1186/s12888-022-04385-3.

Oschatz, Corinna, Jeff Niederdeppe, and Jiawei Liu. 2021. "The Role of Prior Attitudes in Narrative Persuasion: Evidence from a Cross-National Study in Germany and the United States." *Communication Monographs* 89 (3): 376–95. https://doi.org/10.1080/03637751.2021.2011344.

Pabayo, Roman, Claire Benny, and Peter Muennig. 2021. "Financial Barriers to Mental Healthcare Services and Depressive Symptoms Among Residents of Washington Heights, New York City." *Health Promotion Practice* 20 (3): 345–53. https://doi.org/10.1177/15404153211057563.

"Palestinian Radical Denies Link to Flight 103 Bombing." 1990. *New York Times*, January 10, 1990. https://www.nytimes.com/1990/01/10/world/palestinian-radical-denies-link-to-flight-103-bombing.html?searchResultPosition=39.

Park, Sunhee, Haein Lee, and Junghee Kim. 2022. "Role of Alcohol Media Literacy in Alcohol Use among Children and Adolescents: A Systematic Review." *Health Promotion International* 37 (6): daac118. https://doi.org/10.1093/heapro/daac118.

Patte, Karen A., Katelyn Battista, Jessica Goddard, Jordana Ferro, and Scott T. Leatherdale. 2024. "Students' Reasons for Being Reluctant to Seek Help for Mental Health Concerns in Secondary Schools." *Cogent Mental Health* 3 (1): 1–17. https://doi.org/10.1080/28324765.2023.2298918.

Pereira, Sara, and Pedro Moura. 2022. "Assessing Media Literacy Competences: Reflections and Recommendations from a Study with Portuguese Young People." *Journal of Media Literacy Education* 14 (3): 79–93. https://files.eric.ed.gov/fulltext/EJ1373963.pdf.

Pereira, Sara, Manuel Pinto, and Pedro Filipe Ribeiro de Moura. 2015. *Níveis de literacia mediática: estudo exploratório com jovens do 12.º ano* [Levels of Media Literacy: An Exploratory Study with Young People in the 12th Grade]. Centro de Estudos de Comunicação e Sociedade. https://hdl.handle.net/1822/40488.

Philippe, Tristan J., Naureen Sikder, Anna Jackson, Maya E. Koblanski, Eric Liow, Andreas Pilarinos, and Krisztina Vasarhelyi. 2022. "Digital Health Interventions for Delivery of Mental Health Care: Systematic and Comprehensive Meta-Review." *JMIR Mental Health* 9 (5): e35159. https://doi.org/10.2196/35159.

Pimenta, Sofia M., Simon C. Hunter, and Bethany Martin. 2022. "Young People's Coping Strategies When Dealing With Their Own and a Friend's Symptoms of Poor Mental Health: A Qualitative Study." *Journal of Adolescent Research* 39 (3): 375–405. https://doi.org/10.1177/07435584211062115.

Polanco-Levicán, Karina, and Sonia Salvo-Garrido. 2022. "Understanding Social Media Literacy: A Systematic Review of the Concept and Its Competences." *International Journal of Environmental Research and Public Health* 19 (15): 9325204. https://doi.org/10.3390/ijerph19159325.

Potter, W. James. 2004. *Theory of Media Literacy: A Cognitive Approach*. SAGE.

Potter, W. James. 2019. *Media Literacy*, 9th ed. SAGE.

Powell, Kalynda, Elizabeth Huxley, and Michelle L. Townsend. 2021. "Mental Health Help Seeking in Young People and Carers in Out-of-Home Care: A Systematic Review." *Children and Youth Services Review* 129: 106182. https://doi.org/10.1016/j.childyouth.2021.106182.

Pretorius, Claudette, Derek Chambers, and David Coyle. 2019a. "Young People's Online Help-Seeking and Mental Health Difficulties: Systematic Narrative Review." *Journal of Medical Internet Research* 21 (11): e13873. https://doi.org/10.2196/13873.

Pretorius, Claudette, Derek Chambers, Benjamin Cowan, and David Coyle. 2019b. "Young People Seeking Help Online for Mental Health: Cross-Sectional Survey Study." *JMIR Mental Health* 6 (8): e13524. https://doi.org/10.2196/13524.

Pretorius, Claudette, Darragh McCashin, Naoise Kavanagh, and David Coyle. 2020. "Searching for Mental Health: A Mixed Methods Study of Young People's Online Help-Seeking." In *Proceedings of the 2020 CHI Conference on Human Factors in Computing Systems*, 1–13. Honolulu, HI: Association for Computing Machinery. https://doi.org/10.1145/3313831.3376328.

Primack, Brian A., Melissa A. Gold, George E. Switzer, Renee Hobbs, Susan R. Land, and Michael J. Fine. 2006. "Development and Validation of a Smoking Media Literacy Scale for Adolescents." *Archives of Pediatrics and Adolescent Medicine* 160: 360–74. https://doi.org/10.1001/archpedi.160.4.369.

Primack, Jennifer M., Michael E. Addis, Matthew Syzdek, and Ivan W. Miller. 2010. "The Men's Stress Workshop: A Gender-Sensitive Treatment for Depressed Men." *Psychotherapy* 47 (3): 276–87. https://doi.org/10.1016/j.psychotherapy.2009.09.001.

Qazvinian, Vahed, Emily Rosengren, Dragomir R. Radev, and Qiaozhu Mei. 2011. "Rumor Has It: Identifying Misinformation in Microblogs." In *Proceedings of the Conference on Empirical Methods in Natural Language Processing, 2011*, 1589–99. Available at: https://www.aclweb.org/anthology/D11-1147.pdf.

Ramos-Yamamoto, Adriana, and Amy Rose. 2019. *California College Students Are Increasingly Experiencing Mental Health Issues and Need Improved Support.* May 2019. California Budget & Policy Center. https://calbudgetcenter.org/resources/california-college-students-are-increasingly-experiencing-mental-health-issues-and-need-improved-support/.

Reavley, Nicola J., Terence V. McCann, Stefan Cvetkovski, and Anthony F. Jorm. 2014. "A Multifaceted Intervention to Improve Mental Health Literacy in Students of a Multicampus University: A Cluster Randomised Trial." *Social Psychiatry and Psychiatric Epidemiology* 49 (10): 1655–66. https://doi.org/10.1007/s00127-014-0880-6.

Richard, Jérémie, Reid Rebinsky, Rahul Suresh, Serena Kubic, Adam Carter, Jasmyn E. A. Cunningham, Amy Ker, Kayla Williams, and Mark Sorin. 2022. "Scoping Review to Evaluate the Effects of Peer Support on the Mental Health of Young Adults." *BMJ Open* 12 (8): e061336. https://doi.org/10.1136/bmjopen-2022-061336.

Richman, Mike. 2017. "Veterans Face Challenges in Higher Education Not Seen by Other Students." *VA Research Currents*, October 26, 2017. https://www.research.va.gov/currents/1017-Veterans-face-challenges-in-higher-education.cfm.

Rickwood, Debra, Frank P. Deane, Coralie Wilson, and Judy Ciarrochi. 2005. "Young People's Help-Seeking for Mental Health Problems." *Advances in Mental Health* 4 (3): 218–51. https://doi.org/10.5172/jamh.4.3.218.

Rizwan, Bushra, and Paul E. Weigle. 2025. "Paging Dr Influencer: Social Media & Psychiatric Self-Diagnosis." *Pediatric Clinics of North America* 72 (2): 267–78. https://doi.org/10.1016/j.pcl.2024.11.007.

Rogow, Faith. 2009. "Voices from the Field: Teaching Media Literacy in Less Than an Hour." *Journal of Media Literacy Education* 1 (1): 72–3. https://files.eric.ed.gov/fulltext/EJ1095255.pdf.

Romeo, Isabella, Harold Stanislaw, Jamie McCreary, and Marcus Hawley. 2024. "The Importance of Belonging for Well-Being in College Students." *PLOS Mental Health* 1 (1): e0000057. https://doi.org/10.1371/journal.pmen.0000057.

Rothwell, Jonathan. 2023a. "Parenting Mitigates Social Media-Linked Mental Health Issues." *Gallup News*, October 27, 2023. https://news.gallup.com/poll/513248/parenting-mitigates-social-media-linked-mental-health-issues.aspx.

Rothwell, Jonathan. 2023b. "Teens Spend Average of 4.8 Hours on Social Media Per Day." *Gallup News*, October 13, 2023. https://news.gallup.com/poll/512576/teens-spend-average-hours-social-media-per-day.aspx.

Saad, Lydia. 2022. "Americans Have Close but Wary Bond With Their Smartphone." *Gallup News*, June 20, 2022. https://news.gallup.com/poll/393785/americans-close-wary-bond-smartphone.aspx.

Sagar-Ouriaghli, Ilyas, Emma Godfrey, and June S. L. Brown. 2019. "Improving Mental Health Service Utilization Among Men: A Systematic Review and Synthesis of Behavior Change Techniques Within Interventions Targeting Help-Seeking." *American Journal of Men's Health* 13 (3): 1–18. https://doi.org/10.1177/1557988319857009.

Salaheddin, Keziban, and Barbara Mason. 2016. "Identifying Barriers to Mental Health Help-Seeking among Young Adults in the UK: A Cross-Sectional Survey." *British Journal of General Practice* 66 (651): e686–92. https://doi.org/10.3399/bjgp16X687313.

Samuel, Rosalia, and Stuart B. Kamenetsky. 2022. "Help-Seeking Preferences and Factors Associated with Attitudes Toward Seeking Mental Health Services Among First-Year Undergraduates." *Canadian Journal of Higher Education* 52 (1): 31–48. https://files.eric.ed.gov/fulltext/EJ1350851.pdf.

Sandhu, Harman S., Anish Arora, and Jennifer Brasch. 2019. "Correlates of Explicit and Implicit Stigmatizing Attitudes of Canadian Undergraduate University Students toward Mental Illness: A Cross-Sectional Study." *Journal of American College Health* 68 (5): 567–71. https://doi.org/10.1080/07448481.2019.1682002.

Schreurs, Lara, and Laura Vandenbosch. 2021. "Introducing the Social Media Literacy (SMILE) Model with the Case of the Positivity Bias on Social Media." *Journal of Children and Media* 15 (3): 320–37. https://doi.org/10.1080/17482798.2020.1809481.

Schreurs, Lara, Adrian Meier, and Laura Vandenbosch. 2022. "Exposure to the Positivity Bias and Adolescents' Differential Longitudinal Links with Social Comparison, Inspiration, and Envy Depending on Social Media Literacy." *Current Psychology*. https://doi.org/10.1007/s12144-022-03893-3.

Schwartz, Sarah. 2020. "More States Say They're Teaching Media Literacy, but What That Means Varies." *Education Week*, January 8, 2020. https://www.edweek.org/teaching-learning/more-states-say-theyre-teaching-media-literacy-but-what-that-means-varies/2020/01.

Seabrook, Rita C., L. Monique Ward, and Soraya Giaccardi. 2018. "Less Than Human? Media Use, Objectification of Women, and Men's Acceptance of Sexual Aggression." *Psychology of Women Quarterly* 42 (4): 460–76. https://doi.org/10.1177/0361684318795886.

Shandley, Kerrie, David Austin, Britt Klein, and Michael Kyrios. 2010. "An Evaluation of 'Reach Out Central': An Online Gaming Program for Supporting the Mental Health of Young People." *Health Education Research* 25 (4): 563–74. https://doi.org/10.1093/her/cyq002.

Shannon, Holly, Katie Bush, Paul J. Villeneuve, Kim G. C. Hellemans, and Synthia Guimond. 2022. "Problematic Social Media Use in Adolescents and Young Adults: Systematic Review and Meta-Analysis." *JMIR Mental Health* 9 (4): e33450. https://doi.org/10.2196/33450.

Share, Jeff, and Tatevik Mamikonyan. 2020. "Preparing English Teachers with Critical Media Literacy for the Digital Age." *Contemporary Issues in Technology and Teacher Education* 20 (1). https://citejournal.org/volume-20/issue-1-20/english-language-arts/preparing-english-teachers-with-critical-media-literacy-for-the-digital-age/.

Sharpe, Hannah, Priya Patalay, Panos Vostanis, Jay Belsky, Neil Humphrey, and Miranda Wolpert. 2017. "Use, Acceptability, and Impact of Booklets Designed to Support Mental Health Self-Management and Help-Seeking in Schools: Results of a Large Randomised Controlled Trial in England." *European Child & Adolescent Psychiatry* 26: 315–24. https://doi.org/10.1007/s00787-016-0889-3.

Shrivastava, Saurabh R., Prateek S. Shrivastava, and Jegadeesh Ramasamy. 2014. "Enhancing Mental Health Literacy in India to Reduce Stigma: The Fountainhead to Improve Help-Seeking Behaviour." *Journal of Public Mental Health* 13 (3): 159–70. https://doi.org/10.1108/JPMH-06-2013-0043.

Siddique, Md Abu Bakar, Musaddiqur Rahman Ovi, Tanvir Ahammed, Muhammad Abdul Baker Chowdhury, and Md Jamal Uddin. 2022. "Mental Health Knowledge and Awareness Among University Students in Bangladesh." *PLOS ONE* 17 (10): e0269927. https://doi.org/10.1371/journal.pone.0269927.

Sim, Kai Ying H., and Kimberly Tze Wei Choo. 2025. "I Said Things I Needed to Hear Myself: Peer Support as an Emotional, Organisational, and Sociotechnical Practice in Singapore." *arXiv Preprint*, June 11, 2025. https://arxiv.org/abs/2506.09362.

Simons, Mathea, Will Meeus, and Jan T'Sas. 2017. "Measuring Media Literacy for Media Education: Development of a Questionnaire for Teachers' Competencies." *Journal of Media Literacy Education* 9 (1): 99–115. https://doi.org/10.23860/JMLE-2017-9-1-7.

Sitrin, Carly. 2023. "New Jersey Becomes First State to Mandate K-12 Students Learn Information Literacy." *Politico*, January 5, 2023. https://www.politico.com/news/2023/01/05/new-jersey-is-the-first-state-to-mandate-k-12-students-learn-information-literacy-00076352.

Smith, Joshua P., Giao Q. Tran, and Rachel D. Thompson. 2008. "Can the Theory of Planned Behavior Help Explain Men's Psychological Help-Seeking? Evidence for a Mediation Effect and Clinical Implications." *Psychology of Men & Masculinity* 9 (3): 179–92. https://doi.org/10.1037/1524-9220.9.3.179.

Soares, Claudio N., Min Zhang, and Matthieu Boucher. 2019. "Categorical Improvement in Functional Impairment in Depressed Patients Treated with Desvenlafaxine." *Neuropsychiatric Disease and Treatment* 15: 1865–73. https://doi.org/10.2147/NDT.S208070.

Solmi, Marco, Joaquim Radua, Marco Olivola, Eleonora Croce, Luca Soardo, Gonzalo Salazar de Pablo, Jinhee Il Shin, James B. Kirkbride, Peter Jones, Ji Hyun Kim, Jin Yeong Kim, Andre F. Carvalho, Mary V. Seeman, Christoph U. Correll, and Paolo Fusar-Poli. 2022. "Age at Onset of Mental Disorders Worldwide: Large-Scale Meta-Analysis of 192 Epidemiological Studies." *Molecular Psychiatry* 27: 281–95. https://doi.org/10.1038/s41380-021-01161-7.

Sommariva, Silvia, Cheryl Vamos, Alexios Mantzarlis, Lillie Uyên-Loan Đào, and Dinorah Martinez Tyson. 2018. "Spreading the (Fake) News: Exploring Health Messages on Social Media and the Implications for Health Professionals Using a Case Study." *Health Communication* 33 (3): 246–55. https://doi.org/10.1080/19325037.2018.1473178.

Sontag-Padilla, Lisa, Rachana Seelam, Courtney Ann Kase, Michelle W. Woodbridge, and Bradley D. Stein. 2018. "Student Access to Mental Health Information on California College Campuses." *Rand Health Quarterly* 7 (2): 7. https://www.ncbi.nlm.nih.gov/pmc/articles/PMC5798969/.

Spikes, Michael, and Michelle R. Nelson. 2022. "It's the (Unfunded!) Law: How High School Teachers Define & Teach Media Literacy." *Media Education Research*, November 18, 2022. https://mediaeducation.illinois.edu/research/.

Squires, Lauren, Ashley Peters, and Lindsey Rohr. 2023. "Exploring Critical Media Health Literacy (CMHL) in the Online Classroom." *Journal of Media Literacy Education* 15 (1): 58–71. https://doi.org/10.23860/JMLE-2023-15-1-5.

Stepanova, Evgenia, Sarah Croke, Ge Yu, Oládayò Bífárìn, Maria Panagioti, and Yu Fu. 2025. "I Am Not a Priority: Ethnic Minority Experiences of Navigating Mental Health Support and the Need for Culturally Sensitive Services During and Beyond the Pandemic." *BMJ Mental Health* 28 (1): 1–8. https://doi.org/10.1136/bmjment-2024-301481.

Stellefson, Michael, Beth H. Paige, John D. Chaney, and D. Chaney. 2020. "Evolving Role of Social Media in Health Promotion: Updated Responsibilities for Health Education Specialists." *International Journal of Environmental Research and Public Health* 17 (4): 1153. https://doi.org/10.3390/ijerph17041153.

Stretton, Alexander, Barbara A. Spears, Carmel Taddeo, and Judy Drennan. 2018. "Help-Seeking Online by Young People: Does the Influence of Others Matter?" *International Journal of Emotional Education* 10 (1): 95–111. https://files.eric.ed.gov/fulltext/EJ1177656.pdf.

Stunden, Chelsea, Julie Zasada, Nicole VanHeerwaarden, Elisa Hollenberg, Alexxa Abi-Jaoudé, Gloria Chaim, Kristin Cleverley, Joanna Henderson, Andrew Johnson, Andrea Levinson, Brian Lo, Janine Robb, Jenny Shi, Aristotle Voineskos, and David Wiljer. 2020. "Help-Seeking Behaviors of Transition-Aged Youth for Mental Health Concerns: Qualitative Study." *Journal of Medical Internet Research* 22 (10): e18514. https://doi.org/10.2196/18514.

Substance Abuse and Mental Health Services Administration. 2019. *Student Assistance: A Guide for School Administrators.* US Department of Health and Human Services. https://library.samhsa.gov/sites/default/files/tthy-student-assistance-guide-pep19-03-01-001.pdf.

SUNY Empire State College. n.d. "Women, Girls & the Media." *SUNY Online.* Accessed December 20, 2024. https://explore.suny.edu/courses/1338971.

Suwanwong, Charin, Anchalee Jansem, Ungsinun Intarakamhang, Pitchada Prasittichok, Sudarat Tuntivivat, Krittipat Chuenphittayavut, Khuong Le, and Le Thi Mai Lien. 2024. "Modifiable Predictors of Mental Health Literacy in the Educational Context: A Systematic Review and Meta-Analysis." *BMC Psychology* 12: 378. https://doi.org/10.1186/s40359-024-01878-4.

Szabó, Dániel, Krisztina Győri, Péter Lajos, and Gabriella Pusztai. 2024. "Systematic Literature Review on Parental Involvement in Digital Education." *Journal of Media Literacy Education* 16 (2): 98–107. https://doi.org/10.23860/JMLE-2024-16-2-8.

Szabo, Kornelia, Irena Szumska, and Ferenc Túry. 2012. "Media Literacy Programs in the Prevention of Eating Disorders: Potentials, Efficacy, and Limitations." Paper Presented at the 2012 International Congress of Behavioral Medicine, Budapest. https://www.researchgate.net/publication/272998781_Media_literacy_programs_in_the_prevention_of_eating_disorders_Potentials_efficacy_and_limitations.

Talagala, Nisha. 2023. "The AI Literacy Act – What Is It and Why Should You Care?" *Forbes*, December 29, 2023. https://www.forbes.com/sites/nishatalagala/2023/12/29/the-ai-literacy-actwhat-is-it-and-why-should-you-care/?sh=475beca353a4.

Tam, Mallorie T., Julia M. Wu, Cindy C. Zhang, Colleen Pawliuk, and Julie M. Robillard. 2024. "A Systematic Review of the Impacts of Media Mental Health Awareness Campaigns on Young People." *Health Promotion Practice* 25 (5): 907–20. https://doi.org/10.1177/15248399241232646.

Tambling, Rachel R., Carissa D'Aniello, and Beth S. Russell. 2023. "Mental Health Literacy: A Critical Target for Narrowing Racial Disparities in Behavioral Health." *International Journal of Mental Health and Addiction* 21: 1867–81. https://doi.org/10.1007/s11469-021-00694-w.

Tamplin, Natalie C., Siân A. McLean, and Susan J. Paxton. 2018. "Social Media Literacy Protects Against the Negative Impact of Exposure to Appearance Ideal Social Media Images in Young Adult Women but Not Men." *Body Image* 26: 29–37. https://doi.org/10.1016/j.bodyim.2018.05.003.

Tan, X., and Y. Mao. 2023. "Adverse Childhood Experiences and Depression: Do Less Count for More?" *Journal of Affective Disorders* 315: 123–31. https://doi.org/10.1016/j.jad.2022.11.034.

Tang, Yuxi, and Weiguang He. 2023. "Meta-Analysis of the Relationship Between University Students' Anxiety and Academic Performance During the Coronavirus Disease 2019 Pandemic." *Frontiers in Psychology* 14: 1018558. https://doi.org/10.3389/fpsyg.2023.1018558.

Tanner, Joachim, Thomas Zeffiro, Daniela Wyss, Noelle Perron, Michel Rufer, and Christoph Mueller-Pfeiffer. 2019. "Psychiatric Symptom Profiles Predict Functional Impairment." *Frontiers in Psychiatry* 10: 37. https://doi.org/10.3389/fpsyt.2019.00037.

Testa, Michael. 2023. "Testa Sets the Record Straight on New Information Literacy Law." January 6, 2023. https://www.senatenj.com/ArchiveCenter/ViewFile/Item/2244?utm

Thomas, Deja. 2023. "Californians' Mental Health Varies Across Key Groups." *Public Policy Institute of California*. Accessed December 7, 2024. https://www.ppic.org/blog/californians-mental-health-varies-across-key-groups/.

Thomson, Meigan, Gregor Henderson, Tim Rogers, Benjamin Locke, John Vines, and Angus MacBeth. 2024. "Digital Mental Health and Peer Support: Building a Theory of Change Informed by Stakeholders' Perspectives." *PLOS Digital Health* 3 (1): e0000522. https://doi.org/10.1371/journal.pdig.0000522.

Tomczyk, Samuel, Georg Schomerus, Susanne, Stolzenburg, Holger Muehlan, and Silke Schmidt. 2020. "Ready, Willing and Able? An Investigation of the Theory of Planned Behaviour in Help-Seeking for a Community Sample with Current Untreated Depressive Symptoms." *Prevention Science* 21 (6): 749–60. https://doi.org/10.1007/s11121-020-01099-2.

Torous, John, Jennifer Wisniewski, Haiden Bird, and Matcheri S. Keshavan. 2021. "The Growing Field of Digital Psychiatry: Current Evidence and the Future of Apps, Social Media, Chatbots, and Virtual Reality." *World Psychiatry* 20 (3): 318–35. https://doi.org/10.1002/wps.20883.

Tsay-Vogel, Mina. 2015. "Third-Person Effect." In *The International Encyclopedia of Media Effects*, edited by Patrick Rössler, 1–5. Wiley. https://doi.org/10.1002/9781119011071.iemp0130.

Tugtekin, Esra Barut, and Mustafa Koc. 2019. "Understanding the Relationship between New Media Literacy, Communication Skills, and Democratic Tendency: Model Development and Testing." *New Media & Society* 22 (2): 1922–41. https://doi.org/10.1177/1461444819887705.

Turin, Ornat, and Yonty Friesem. 2020. "Is That Media Literacy?: Israeli and US Media Scholars' Perceptions of the Field." *Journal of Media Literacy Education* 12 (1). https://digitalcommons.uri.edu/jmle/vol12/iss1/10/.

Twenge, Jean M., Thomas E. Joiner, Megan L. Rogers, and Gabrielle N. Martin. 2018. "Increases in Depressive Symptoms, Suicide-Related Outcomes, and Suicide Rates Among US Adolescents After 2010 and Links to Increased New Media Screen Time." *Clinical Psychological Science* 6 (1): 3–17. https://doi.org/10.1177/2167702617723376.

UCLA Library. n.d. "Education 466: Media Literacy." Accessed December 19, 2024. https://guides.library.ucla.edu/educ466.

United Nations Office on Drugs and Crime. 2021. "Good Use and Abuse: The Role of Technology in Human Trafficking." Accessed December 8, 2024. https://www.unodc.org/unodc/en/human-trafficking/Webstories2021/the-role-of-technology-in-human-trafficking.html.

US Census Bureau. n.d. "QuickFacts: Valley Center CDP, California." Accessed December 13, 2024. https://www.census.gov/quickfacts/valleycentercdpcalifornia.

US Congress. 2022. *S.4490 - Digital Citizenship and Media Literacy Act.* Introduced by Sen. Amy Klobuchar [D-MN], June 23, 2022. https://www.congress.gov/bill/117th-congress/senate-bill/4490.

US Congress. 2023. *H.R. 6791 - Artificial Intelligence Literacy Act of 2023.* Introduced by Rep. Lisa Blunt Rochester [D-DE-At Large], December 14, 2023. https://www.congress.gov/bill/118th-congress/house-bill/6791.

US Department of State. 2021. "Media 4 Women: A Media Literacy Program for Vulnerable Groups." *State Alumni*, October 26, 2021. https://alumni.state.gov/highlight/media-4-women-media-literacy-program-vulnerable-groups.

Verswijvel, Karen, Michel Walrave, Kris Hardies, and Wannes Heirman. 2019. "Sharenting, Is It a Good or a Bad Thing? Understanding How Adolescents Think and Feel about Sharenting on Social Network Sites." *Children and Youth Services Review* 104: 104401. https://doi.org/10.1016/j.childyouth.2019.104401.

Villatoro, Alice P., Melissa J. DuPont-Reyes, Jo C. Phelan, and Bruce G. Link. 2023. "'Me' vs. 'Them': How Mental Illness Stigma Influences Adolescent Help-Seeking Behaviors for Oneself and Recommendations for Peers." *Stigma and Health* 8 (1): 13–25. https://doi.org/10.1037/sah0000446.

Vine, Vera, Ryan L. Boyd, and James W. Pennebaker. 2020. "Natural Emotion Vocabularies as Windows on Distress and Well-Being." *Nature Human Behaviour* 4: 1025–35. https://doi.org/10.1038/s41562-020-0906-4.

Vogels, Emily A. 2022. "Teens and Cyberbullying 2022." *Pew Research Center*, December 15, 2022. https://www.pewresearch.org/internet/2022/12/15/teens-and-cyberbullying-2022/.

Vogels, Emily A., and Risa Gelles-Watnick. 2023. "Teens and Social Media: Key Findings from Pew Research Center Surveys." *Pew Research Center*, April 24, 2023.

https://www.pewresearch.org/short-reads/2023/04/24/teens-and-social-media-key-findings-from-pew-research-center-surveys/.

Wade, Tracey D., Susan Davidson, and Jennifer A. O'Dea. 2003. "A Preliminary Controlled Evaluation of a School-Based Media Literacy Program and Self-Esteem Program for Reducing Eating Disorder Risk Factors." *International Journal of Eating Disorders* 33 (4): 371–83. https://doi.org/10.1002/eat.10136.

Walter, Nathan, John J. Brooks, Camille J. Saucier, and Sapna Suresh. 2021. "Evaluating the Impact of Attempts to Correct Health Misinformation on Social Media: A Meta-Analysis." *Health Communication* 35 (14): 1776–84. https://doi.org/10.1080/10410236.2020.1794553.

Walton, Gregory M., Mary C. Murphy, Christine Logel, David S. Yeager, J. Parker Goyer, Shannon T. Brady, Katherine T. U. Emerson, David Paunesku, Omid Fotuhi, and Natasha Krol. 2023. "Where and with Whom Does a Brief Social-Belonging Intervention Promote Progress in College?" *Science* 381 (6657): eade4420. https://doi.org/10.1126/science.ade4420.

Wang, Huan, Cody Abbey, Thomas Kennedy, Erik Feng, Robin Li, Finley Liu, Annli Zhu, Sharon Shen, Prateek Wadhavkar, Scott Rozelle, and Manpreet K. Singh. 2023. "The Association Between Screen Time and Outdoor Time on Adolescent Mental Health and Academic Performance: Evidence from Rural China." *International Journal of Environmental Research and Public Health* 20 (5): 4377. https://doi.org/10.3390/ijerph20054377.

Wang, Kira, Nomi Werner-Seidler, Erin E. Michalak, and Janis L. Whitlock. 2022. "Barriers to Mental Health Treatment Among Young Adults With Depression: A US Population-Based Study." *JAMA Network Open* 5 (5): e2212319. https://doi.org/10.1001/jamanetworkopen.2022.12319.

Weinstein, Emily, and Carrie James. 2022. "School-Based Initiatives Promoting Digital Citizenship and Healthy Digital Media Use." In *The Handbook of Adolescent Digital Media Use and Mental Health*, edited by Jacqueline Nesi, Eva H. Telzer, and Mitchell J. Prinstein. Cambridge University Press. https://doi.org/10.1017/9781108976237.

Weiss, Margaret D., Nicole Michelle McBride, Stephanie Craig, and Peter Jensen. 2018. "Conceptual Review of Measuring Functional Impairment: Findings from the Weiss Functional Impairment Rating Scale." *Canadian Journal of Psychiatry* 63 (12): 804–14. https://doi.org/10.1177/0706743718760291.

Wiener, Jocelyn. 2019. "Breakdown: California's Mental Health System, Explained." *CalMatters*, August 23, 2019. https://calmatters.org/explainers/breakdown-californias-mental-health-system-explained/.

Westberg, Maria, Maria Nyholm, Jens M. Nygren, and Petra Svedberg. 2022. "Mental Health Problems Among Young People—A Scoping Review of Help-Seeking." *International Journal of Environmental Research and Public Health* 19 (3): 1430. https://doi.org/10.3390/ijerph19031430.

Wharf Higgins, Joan, and Deborah Begoray. 2012. "Exploring the Borderlands between Media and Health: Conceptualizing 'Critical Media Health Literacy'." *Journal of Media Literacy Education* 4 (2): 136–48. https://digitalcommons.uri.edu/jmle/vol4/iss2/3.

World Health Organization. 2022. "COVID-19 Pandemic Triggers 25% Increase in Prevalence of Anxiety and Depression Worldwide." March 2, 2022. https://www.who.int/news/item/02-03-2022-covid-19-pandemic-triggers-25-increase-in-prevalence-of-anxiety-and-depression-worldwide.

Wright, Annemarie, Anthony F. Jorm, and Andrew J. Mackinnon. 2012. "Labels Used by Young People to Describe Mental Disorders: Which Ones Predict Effective Help-Seeking Choices?" *Social Psychiatry and Psychiatric Epidemiology* 47 (6): 917–26. https://doi.org/10.1007/s00127-011-0399-z.

Wright, Michaela, Franziska Reitegger, Herald Cela, Andrea Papst, and Barbara Gasteiger-Klicpera. 2023. "Interventions with Digital Tools for Mental Health Promotion among 11–18 Year Olds: A Systematic Review and Meta-Analysis." *Journal of Youth and Adolescence* 52 (4): 754–79. https://doi.org/10.1007/s10964-023-01735-4.

Wriston, Blair, Nancy Duchesneau, and Manny Zapata. 2023. *How Mental Health Supports Impact Social, Emotional, and Academic Development (SEAD)*. The Education Trust. https://edtrust.org/rti/how-mental-health-supports-impact-social-emotional-and-academic-development-sead/.

Xin, Meiqi, Sitong Luo, and Joseph Tak-Fai Lau. 2022. "The Roles of Information Valence, Media Literacy, and Perceived Information Quality on the Association Between Frequent Social Media Exposure and COVID-19 Vaccination Intention." *American Journal of Health Promotion* 37 (2): 189–99. https://doi.org/10.1177/08901171221121292.

Yildiz Durak, Hatice, and Mustafa Saritepeci. 2019. "Modeling the Effect of New Media Literacy Levels and Social Media Usage Status on Problematic Internet Usage Behaviours among High School Students." *Education and Information Technologies* 24 (4): 2205–23. https://doi.org/10.1007/s10639-019-09864-9.

Yirenya-Tawiah, Abena and Catherine Cubbin. 2025. "Racial and Ethnic Disparities in Mental Health Service Utilization During COVID-19." *Journal of Racial and Ethnic Health Disparities*: 1–9. https://doi.org/10.1007/s40615-025-02456-z.

Yousaf, Omar, Aneka Popat, and Myra S. Hunter. 2015. "An Investigation of Masculinity Attitudes, Gender, and Attitudes Toward Psychological Help-Seeking." *Psychology of Men and Masculinity* 16 (2): 234–7. https://doi.org/10.1037/a0036241.

YouthTruth. 2024. *Students Weigh In, Part IV*. Accessed December 13, 2024. https://youthtruth.org/wp-content/uploads/2024/05/YouthTruth-Students-Weigh-In-Part-IV.pdf.

Zhang, Jianwu, Chun Peng, and Chen Chen. 2024. "Mental Health and Academic Performance of College Students: Knowledge in the Field of Mental Health, Self-

Control, and Learning in College." *Acta Psychologica* 241: 103042. https://doi.org/10.1016/j.actpsy.2024.103042.

Zhou, Jia, Jingjing Zhou, Lei Feng, Yuan Feng, Le Xiao, Xu Chen, Jian Yang, and Gang Wang. 2022. "The Associations between Depressive Symptoms, Functional Impairment, and Quality of Life in Patients with Major Depression: Undirected and Bayesian Network Analyses." *Frontiers in Psychiatry* 14: 10600944. https://doi.org/10.3389/fpsyt.2023.10600944.

Zorrilla, Márcia Mónica, Naomi Modeste, Peter C. Gleason, Diadrey-Anne Sealy, Jim E. Banta, and Sang Leng Trieu. 2019. "Depression and Help-Seeking Intention Among Young Adults: The Theory of Planned Behavior." *American Journal of Health Education* 50 (4): 236–44. https://doi.org/10.1080/19325037.2019.1616014.

Index

About the Author

Dr. Jesse Scaccia is the social justice journalism professor in the Media, Communications and Journalism Department at Fresno State University, where he teaches media literacy and journalism, and has taught multiple semesters in Fresno State's bachelor's program at Valley State Prison and Central California Women's Facility. His journalism has been published in the *New York Times*, the *Virginian-Pilot*, the *San Diego Union-Tribune*, the *Coloradoan*, *RVA Magazine*, and the *Fresno Bee*, and he was the executive director for a documentary series on Black Entertainment Television. His work as a community organizer and activist has included being part of land back movements in Colorado, the development of arts districts, successful cannabis law reform movements, and Pride events in Virginia, as well as working full-time at a home for young men in Cape Town, South Africa. He earned a PhD from Colorado State University, an MFA in nonfiction writing from Old Dominion University, and an MA in journalism from New York University.

www.ingramcontent.com/pod-product-compliance
Ingram Content Group UK Ltd.
Pitfield, Milton Keynes, MK11 3LW, UK
UKHW020209290926
15470UKWH00001B/95

9 781666 965094